Personal Change and Reconstruction

Personal Change and Reconstruction

Research on a Treatment of Stuttering

FAY FRANSELLA

Royal Free Hospital School of Medicine, University of London, London, England

1972

ACADEMIC PRESS: London and New York

ACADEMIC PRESS INC. (LONDON) LTD.
24/28 Oval Road
London NW1

United States Edition published by
ACADEMIC PRESS INC.
111 Fifth Avenue
New York, New York 10003

Library of Congress Catalog Card Number: 72–84361
ISBN: 0–12–266150–8

Text set in 11/12 pt. Monotype Old Style, printed by letterpress, and bound in
Great Britain at The Pitman Press, Bath

PREFACE

The title of this book is not what it was originally. In several references to it during preparation it was called "Construct Theory Psychotherapy and Stuttering" followed by the enigmatic "in press" (meaning that it was somewhere between an idea and an accomplished fact).

The problem was two-fold. It was a terrible title, but at the same time it was a title that truly reflected the contents. This book is indeed about personal construct theory (George Kelly), psychotherapy and stuttering. It cuts across these three areas of academic and applied interest—the latter two having built up a vast body of work.

Personal construct theory is a psychological approach to the understanding of man and suggests that he is best seen as an inquirer, a seeker, an experimenter. His aim is to interpret events in his environment and to predict future events so as to gain some control over them—thus imposing structure and meaning onto the things that happen to him.

Stuttering is seen as being the person's way of interpreting and thereby exerting some control over his life of inter-personal communication. This world of communication he knows and he will not change this until the world of communicating as a fluent speaker seems at least as meaningful to him. It is no easier for the stutterer to act the fluent speaker than it would be for you or me to adopt the psychological posture of a person of the opposite sex.

Treatment was focused on increasing the meaningfulness of being fluent. Twenty stutterers were treated along the lines suggested by the theory and measurements of speech disfluencies and "meaningfulness" were made at intervals. In an attempt to give the "feel" of the therapeutic approach, massive sections from tape-recorded sessions with one stutterer are presented. Only in this way does it seem possible to convey an idea of how the theory was applied to the treatment of stuttering.

To assist the selective reader, the book is divided into sections. Section I is about some of the things that are known or not known about stuttering and the attempts that have been made to treat it. Section II contains a description of the theoretical approach and Section III is a report of the results of the research. The remaining two sections cover the verbatim accounts of some of the treatment sessions with one stutterer and ideas of research possibilities into the treatment of stuttering and other psychological disorders following the same theoretical lines.

July, 1972.   FAY FRANSELLA

FOREWORD

Most original books in psychology (as distinct from textbooks and textbook re-hashes of textbooks) can be slotted into one of three categories. There are books expounding a particular theory or approach (Schnechwaggenhammer's "A Diagonal Approach to Psychology"); books reporting experimental research (Hammerschneckenwagger's "A Questionnaire Investigation of Secrecy"); or books assembling a multiplicity of material on single topics (Waggenhammerschnecken's "Sex"). It could be that readers as well as books are so categorized.

This book is oddly comprehensive in that it exemplifies a theory (personal construct theory) by reporting a novel piece of experimental work appropriate to the theory on a traditional topic of absorbing interest—stuttering.

It will be interesting to see whether this trinity of ventures in one book trebles its audience or makes it universally indigestible. Personally I like the combination because it convinces me that the author takes her approach seriously. It is one thing to applaud a theoretical framework in print. It is quite another to invest many hundreds of hours of experimental psychotherapy in testing its usefulness. Additionally the spectacle of a theory being made to work for its living—as distinct from providing valid mini-hypotheses for neat little journal papers—is intriguing.

The particular explanation given for the persistence of stuttering is valuable because it provides a mode of attack on the problem for the stutterer and the therapist. It is equally valuable because it is a kind of *explanation* which can be applied to many other personal problems.

Of the book as a whole I can pay it the highest compliment any book can be paid, by saying—read it.

D. BANNISTER

ACKNOWLEDGEMENTS

So many people have helped in the development of this book that it is hard to know with whom to start. Perhaps I should single out Luke. He helped in so many ways, both with and without awareness. Certainly, without him and the permission he gave for vast sections of our sessions together to be published, the book would be divest of any sense of human involvement. Next I must express my gratitude to those who were involved in typing the many drafts, particularly Edith Watson, Susan Sainsbury and Gayle Ginnings. Mrs. Ginnings also performed the laborious task of categorizing all the constructs elicited from the group.

To Dr. D. Bannister, my lasting thanks; primarily for his constant encouragement, but also for reading through all the transcripts of more than eighty tape-recorded therapy sessions with Luke and commenting upon them and for reading the final draft and making many constructive suggestions.

Finally, I am most grateful to the Mental Health Research Fund for granting me a full-time Personal Research Award to carry out this investigation.

CONTENTS

Section I
STUTTERING

Section II
THEORY

Section I

Stuttering

demonstrable when more discriminating analyses of disfluencies are used.

Diagnosis of stuttering in the adult is a relatively easy matter when compared with diagnosis in the child. If an adult's speech contains seemingly "involuntary, audible or silent, repetitions or prolongations in the utterance of short speech elements, namely: sounds, syllables, and words of one syllable", if he says this speech pattern has been with him for as long as he can remember, if he wants to be rid of it, and if he calls himself a stutterer, he will be diagnosed as such. If he says this speech pattern developed in more recent times, then there may well be some psychological or physical disorder of which this disrupted speech is a direct result.

The only other differential diagnosis that might be made is that of cluttering. This is characterized by very rapid, uncontrollable speech, resulting in truncated, dysrhythmic and sometimes incoherent utterance. This is not a common complaint, but one man in the research to be reported was so diagnosed. There is evidence, based on EEG findings, that cluttering may have neurological origins (Moravek and Langova 1962).

Incidence and Prevalence

Stuttering is far more common in children than in adults, indicating that there are many people who used to stutter and have now grown out of it or overcome it. Andrews and Harris (1964) report that 4·8% of a sample of British adults attending their general practitioners said they used to stutter and 3·6% said there was a family member who stuttered.

Sheehan and Martyn (1970) checked on 5,138 students entering three universities in California (in 1964, 1965 and 1967) and found that four out of five of those who reported having been stutterers as children were no longer having any such problem, and had apparently recovered spontaneously. But these authors did find that every "stuttering" child does not seem to have an equal chance of recovering spontaneously. From their data they were able to estimate that 87% of mild, 75% of moderate and only 50% of severe stuttering children will cease to stutter as they get older.

Andrews and Harris reported that, taking children up to the age of seven in a sample of one thousand, 4% stuttered or had speech hesitancies. But taking the sample as a whole, approximately 3% had stuttered for six months or more. It is possible to generalize the findings about the presence of stuttering in children by saying that the more the sample includes older children the lower the percentage of stutterers found.

The studies reporting incidence of stuttering among school children have been reviewed by Bloodstein (1969) who concludes that it is around 1% in Europe and somewhat less in the United States. The prevalence of stuttering among adult populations is virtually unknown but is probably well below the one in a hundred reported in many samples of children. Van Riper (1971) concludes by saying that "we feel that the literature, miserable as most of it is, indicates clearly that the total *incidence* of stuttering probably amounts conservatively to about 4 per cent of the general population, and that its *prevalence* is highest in pre-school years declining thereafter to an unstable value of less than 1 per cent".

Age of Onset

There is a measure of agreement among the findings concerning the age at which stuttering in children first appears in "diagnosable" form. Nearly all are probably so labelled by the age of nine. Andrews and Harris, for instance, found that 95% had begun to stutter by the age of seven and Morley (1957) reports a figure of 50% by age five. There is also some link between severity and age of onset; the more severe the problem, the earlier it is noted (Andrews and Harris, 1964).

Intelligence and Stuttering

It has often been thought that stuttering is found among more intelligent rather than among less intelligent people, but most surveys provide no evidence to support this belief (e.g. Goodstein, 1958). In fact, one of the surveys (Andrews and Harris, 1964) found that a group of stuttering children had an average IQ seven points *lower* than a non-stuttering group. Williams and his colleagues (1969) demonstrated that a hundred stutterers in the sixth grade at school in the United States of America were significantly retarded academically when compared with three hundred nonstuttering children. However, "the fact that the range of scores is approximately the same for both groups indicates that this finding is not necessarily true for any individual sixth grade stutterer, whose score may place him anywhere from the top to the bottom of the total range of scores". Further evidence led them to conclude that the stuttering child tends to "catch up" academically with the nonstutterer by the eighth grade. They found also that there was no difference in the children's verbal as compared with their non-verbal intellectual level.

The most probable reason for this false belief in the higher intellectual level of the stutterer lies in the fact that in past years the more intelligent person was more likely to seek treatment or, perhaps of even greater importance, was more likely to be able to pay for such treatment.

At the other end of the intellectual scale, the prevalence of stuttering has been reported as being higher among the intellectually subnormal than among the general population. Schlanger and Gottsleben (1957), for instance, found that 17% of a group of five hundred subnormal children stuttered. But this again looks as if it can be attributed to causes other than subnormality itself. In two recent studies no more stuttering was found among subnormal populations than among the general population (Sheehan *et al.*, 1968; Martyn *et al.*, 1969). These authors suggest that the main reason for these discrepant findings lies in the categorizing or diagnosing of speech defects in these abnormal populations.

Sex and Stuttering

One of the very few generalizations that can be made about stuttering with any degree of confidence is that it is more often to be found in males than in females. Not only this but, after reviewing the literature, Schuell (1946) came to the conclusion that the defect was more likely to be severe in males than in females. The general opinion is that male stutterers outnumber female stutterers by about three to one. Both neurological and environmental factors are cited to account for this state of affairs. Johnson favours the cultural explanation, seeing parents as more prone to react unfavourably to disfluent speech in boys than in girls. Goldman (1965) argues in support of this theory that the incidence among Southern negroes, with a matriarchal society, is only 2 to 1 compared with 5 to 1 among white children. However, against this goes Eisenson's interesting data about stuttering in children living in kibbutzim in Israel (1966). These included the finding that "stuttering is found among kibbutzim children who are brought up in a child-oriented setting in at least the same incidence as among children in the United States".

One possible constitutional factor is the fact that girls are more advanced in verbal ability in childhood than boys. They tend to develop speech earlier and to be generally more verbally fluent. Indeed Ssikorski is quoted as having speculated on this point in 1894.

> Owing to hereditary peculiarities the motor centres of a woman's left cerebral hemisphere (which contains the organ of Broca, the centre of speech) develop, generally speaking more quickly than a man's and seem, thanks to a more accomplished structure of certain parts of the brain, less exposed to injuries than those of boys. This accounts not only for the earlier development of speech with girls, but also for other psycho-motor specialities of women, viz: their skill in dancing, singing, and needlework. (Appelt, 1911.)

Socio-economic Factors and Stuttering

Andrews and Harris (1964) found no relationship between social class and stuttering in eighty English stutterers compared with eighty control children. However, among a sample of three hundred and fifty Scottish stuttering children, Morgenstern (1956) had previously found a significant tendency for them to come from the homes of skilled and semi-skilled parents and to be significantly less likely to come from homes in which the parents were classified as unskilled. He suggested that this was in line with Johnson's argument that parents who put emphasis on the rapid achievement of fluency were those who were more likely to have stuttering children; the parents have social aspirations. This would be in line with evidence supporting the conclusion that the more industrialized a society is, with a consequent emphasis on upward social mobility, the greater will be the number of stutterers in that society (e.g. Stewart, 1960; Aron, 1962; Lemert, 1962).

Conclusions

From the foregoing outline of research findings it seems fair to conclude that there is still a great deal to learn about the form of speech classified as stuttering. No attempt has been made to discuss views on the way in which stuttering develops or the various theories that have to do with the cause(s) of stuttering. Detailed reviews can be found in Beech and Fransella (1968), Bloodstein (1969) and Van Riper (1971). What can be concluded is that there is no precise agreement among experts as to the definition of stuttering; that stuttering is difficult to diagnose in the young child, and that the majority of children who start their speaking life with what sounds like stuttering become fluent speakers spontaneously, leaving something less than 1% of the population to go on into adulthood as stutterers. Once an adult, the chances of spontaneous recovery are greatly reduced.

If anything, stutterers as a group may be below average in intelligence rather than above as is commonly thought, but it is more likely they have a range of intelligence comparable to that of the general population. Stutterers are more likely to be men than women, boys than girls. It is possible that there is a relationship between stuttering and social class in industrialized societies, perhaps because of the emphasis on "keeping up with the Jones's".

Still to be discussed is the question of whether stutterers have sufficient psychological characteristics in common for them to be considered as members of a single group or not and in what ways, if any, they differ from nonstutterers other than in their speech.

II. The Stutterer

On coming face to face with a stutterer, there is a moment's discomfort while one adjusts his unspoken "summing-up" system to include the category *a stutterer*. Research findings do seem to suggest that the majority of people carry around with them a stereotype about stutterers, just as they do about national and racial groups. By calling a person *a stutterer* one implies that certain personality or physical characteristics—or both—go hand-in-hand with stuttering. The mere fact that one talks of *a stutterer* instead of *someone who stutters* shows this to be so. A person who lisps is not often called *a lisper* nor a person who limps *a limper*.

Psychologists and speech pathologists also follow this line of thought. For many decades they have sought to uncover the psychological and physiological factors that go along with stuttering and thus make up *the stutterer*. Attempts to describe him and so set him apart from the rest of mankind can very broadly be divided into those seeking (a) to isolate some physical defect that may result from or else cause his stuttering, and (b) to ascribe to him neurotic or other distinguishing personality characteristics. No attempt has been made here to provide an exhaustive coverage of all the work that has been done, but rather it is intended to give an idea of the variety of ways people have thought stutterers *might* differ from nonstutterers.

A. THE PHYSICAL AND CONSTITUTIONAL CHARACTERISTICS OF THE STUTTERER

Most of the systems of the body have either been held responsible for the stutterers' plight or have been implicated as accessories after the fact in setting the stutterer apart from his fellow men. The bodily systems so investigated include the cardiovascular, muscular, respiratory, auditory and nervous, with metabolism thrown in for good measure. Under the general heading of "constitutional factors" can be included investigations into whether changing a child's handedness is related to stuttering; the effects of preventing the stutterer from immediately hearing the sound of his own voice, and the relationship between rhythmic speech and stuttering.

The Cardiovascular System

In a paper entitled "Chemical Factors and the Stuttering Spasm", Johnson *et al.* (1933) examined the blood of fifteen stutterers, varying in age from nine to twenty-eight years, and took measures of serum calcium, potassium, inorganic phosphorus and blood sugar. They thought that, since stuttering was characterized by muscular spasm, there might be an association with latent tetany (tonic contraction, mainly of muscles of the hands and feet, with hypersensitivity of other muscles). The authors found that all their measurements fell within normal limits.

Kopp (1934), however, was not satisfied with this and the following year reported comparing the blood chemistry of a group of stutterers with his own selected group of nonstutterers, concluding that there were considerable *differences* between the blood patterns of the two groups.

Karlin and Sorbel (1940) then proceeded to point out flaws in Kopp's work which could have produced the differences reported, but which have nothing to do with stuttering; for instance Kopp used a group of nonstutterers who differed in age from the group of stutterers. They point out that

> Since it is known that the serum inorganic phosphorus in children is higher than in adults, to assign any significance to higher values in a lower age group other than that of normal variation is not justifiable. (Karlin and Sorbel, 1940.)

To counteract this objection and what they considered to be some other methodological and statistical weaknesses in Kopp's work, Karlin and Sorbel conducted their own research. Their measures all fell within the normal range—there were no statistically significant differences between the blood pattern of the stutterers and nonstutterers.

Similarly, investigators have failed to find any differences in heart rate or general functioning of the heart between stutterers and nonstutterers. Differences that have been observed are readily explicable as resulting from general body activity, especially that occurring during the stuttering act itself.

The Muscular System

Rotter (1955) found that his group of stutterers were less skilled at sorting cards than were nonstutterers when using either the left *or* the right hand, but were equally as skilful when using both hands. But this is one of the very few pieces of research that has found stutterers differing from nonstutterers in motor capabilities.

The contradictory evidence has at times been of quite an extreme nature. For instance, Kopp (1943) gave a test of motor proficiency to four hundred and fifty stutterers and found that the

> motor disturbances are so significant that reversing the classic proposition, we may say that stuttering is not a psychologic disorder; it is first and above all a neurologic disorder characterized by profound disturbance of the motor function.

These findings were so unusual and so at variance with the majority view that Finkelstein and Weisberger (1954) repeated the research. They used only fifteen stutterers but, unlike Kopp, tested a group of nonstutterers matched for age, sex and handedness. No significant differences between the two groups emerged. In fact, the stutterers were actually *in advance* of the nonstutterers in terms of motor age.

Not surprisingly, several people have been concerned with demonstrating that the stutterer has more difficulty in moving and using the muscles and organs concerned in the production of speech. But again, stutterers seem to have tongue strength equal to nonstutterers as well as equally good muscle control of jaw, tongue and lips. Cross (1936) did find that stutterers were slower than nonstutterers in making repetitive movements of the lips, tongue and jaw, but this was contradicted by Spriestersbach (1940) who did not.

While studying the voluntary movements of stutterers, Blackburn (1931) reported that they were markedly inferior to nonstutterers in executing rhythmical voluntary movements of the tongue and diaphragm, but had no great difficulty in performing such movements with other structures concerned with speech. Likewise, Hunsley (1937) found that stutterers did less well with every muscle group when they were required to produce a rhythmic pattern of clicks. There have been several other investigations whose results support this notion of a rhythmical defect. However, there have equally been studies that have produced results showing there to be no such differences. Some have even demonstrated stutterers to be *superior* to nonstutterers in the production of certain rhythmical movements.

There has been particular interest in rhythm because of its ability to produce a marked reduction in stuttering. The great majority of stutterers can utter words without stuttering if they can introduce some degree of rhythmicity into their speech. The imposing of rhythm on the speech, be it by reciting poetry, singing or following the beat of a metronome, produces a flow of speech relatively unbroken by disfluencies. The stutterer can speak without stuttering, but he is still communicating in an abnormal way. There is no evidence to suggest that the conscious use of rhythmic speech rectifies some physiological defect in the stutterer. The most commonly given explanation has been in terms of a distraction. It is suggested that the imposing of rhythm on the speech diverts the stutterer's attention away from the sound of his own voice. Experiments designed to test this idea have consistently produced negative results (e.g. Fransella, 1965; Fransella and Beech, 1965; Fransella, 1967; Brady, 1969).

One other explanation tested (Beech and Fransella, 1969; Fransella, 1971) is that rhythm effectively reduces stuttered speech because it serves to "tell" the stutterer when to say the next word. In support of this idea is the ample evidence that most stuttering occurs on initial word sounds, and the first words of sentences and paragraphs (e.g. Quarrington *et al.*, 1962; Taylor, 1966a). Although some experimental support was found for this hypothesis it was clearly not the complete answer.

An alternative explanation can be found in the fact that rhythmic speech may almost eliminate stuttering, but it does not produce normal fluency. The speech is artificial. One abnormal way of speaking is being exchanged for another. Stuttering, however, is "normal" for the stutterer. Rhythmic speech, like the assumption of a foreign accent, may provide a situation for the stutterer in which he can be someone other than himself which, in turn, often enables him to be stutter-free.

The Respiratory System

Early on in this century several people were recording abnormalities of breathing patterns of stutterers (e.g. Halle, 1900; Travis, 1927). In the normal speaker, chest and abdominal breathing are closely linked, but in the stutterer they were found to be antagonistic to each other. Following another line of inquiry, Starr (1922) described four sub-groups of stutterers, which included sub-breathers, who are "organisms overloaded with carbon-dioxide". Later Van Riper (1936) made the interesting observation that not only were there breathing abnormalities during the actual occurrence of stuttering but that they were also there when the person was *expecting* to stutter.

There is thus ample evidence that the breathing of stutterers is abnormal. But these abnormalities are not found in all of them and every stutterer does not have the same type of breathing abnormality. The main controversy centres around whether stuttering is responsible for bad breathing, or whether bad breathing is responsible for stuttering. It is, however, not too clear from the evidence whether the stutterer has faulty breathing in the speaking *and* the non-speaking situation. If he does, then clearly there is some justification for the many therapeutic programmes that involve exercises in breath control.

Metabolism

As well as finding certain differences in the blood pattern of stutterers and nonstutterers Kopp (1934) concluded that "stuttering is a manifestation of a disturbed metabolism". But once again his findings were not successfully repeated.

It has also been reported that stutterers have a higher hydrogen ion concentration than normal individuals (Kelly, 1932; Starr, 1928), which has been interpreted as indicating that stutterers have too much carbon dioxide in their blood due to inefficient breathing. As with so many other "positive" findings, other workers failed to come up with the same answers (Hill, 1944; Johnson *et al.*, 1959).

McCrosky (1957) failed to find any difference in basal metabolic rate between stutterers and nonstutterers, in either the speaking or the non-speaking situation. Likewise, there is no firm evidence that stuttering is related to endocrine malfunctioning. There have been one or two reports concerning the onset of stuttering in previous nonstutterers who had been given thyroid extract. But even when this occurred, there is doubt as to whether the speech non-fluencies should have been classified as stuttering. In all the reports the "stuttering speech" seems to have stopped when the extract was stopped.

The Nervous System

Investigations in this area have been mainly concerned with whether stutterers have different patterns of electrical activity in the brain compared with nonstutterers. Walter (1961) has graphically described these electroencephalographic (EEG) recordings as follows:

> The electrical changes which give rise to the alternating currents of variable frequency and amplitude thus recorded arise in the cells of the brain itself; there is no question of any other power supply. The brain must be pictured as a vast aggregation of electrical cells, as numerous as the stars of the Galaxy, some ten thousand million of them, through which surge the restless tides of our electrical being relatively thousands of times more potent than the force of gravity. It is when a million or so of these cells repeatedly fire together that the rhythm of their discharge becomes measurable in frequency and amplitude. (Walter, 1961, p. 60.)

Once again the literature on this topic gives conflicting information and results. For instance, Andrews and Harris (1964) investigated thirty pairs of stuttering and nonstuttering children to see whether there was any neurological abnormality connected with their stuttering. Experts, who were in ignorance of the owner of the EEG record, failed to find any differences between the records of the stutterers and the nonstutterers. However, in an investigation using adults (Sayles, 1967), the stutterers had significantly more abnormal EEG tracings than did a comparable group of nonstutterers. There have been a large number of studies yielding such conflicting results. But taking an overall view of the position one can fairly conclude that brain recordings of stutterers *as a group* are normal.

Some of the most interesting studies have been concerned with the question of laterality or cerebral dominance. The fact that most people "favour" one side of the body rather than the other, reflects the fact that one hemisphere of the brain tends to be dominant over the other. It was argued by Orton (1927) and Travis (1931) that, since the muscular movements producing speech involve both sides of the brain, there may be conflict between the two hemispheres if there is a lack of dominance of one side over the other.

The cerebral dominance theory of stuttering provided the fertile soil for one of the most widely held beliefs about stuttering today. The belief that a child will develop a stutter if he is made to change from using his left hand, which he prefers, to his right. It was argued that by doing this the cerebral dominance was disturbed and the resulting conflict or confusion between the two hemispheres led to stuttering. The popularity of this belief has waned little since it arose in the nineteen-twenties, even though Travis himself abandoned the theory in the nineteen-forties because of lack of supporting evidence. In any case the majority of stutterers are right-handed and it seems likely that for every one who was made to change hands and did stutter there is one who changed hands and did *not* develop a stutter.

Some of the irritability arising over the persistence of this belief can be seen in the following passage:

> Thus, the results on all three of the supposed predisposing factors—familial incidence, handedness, and handedness in the family background—were uniformly sterile . . . In planning the study, these items were included with considerable reluctance, for they occupied time and space that might have been devoted to more promising variables. However, the resistance of the dysphemia concept to scientific extinction has been such that it appeared that these data should be gathered. (Sheehan and Martyn, 1966.)

It would seem that both expert and layman have difficulty in ridding themselves of this false belief.

However, before this whole question of the relationship of dominance to stuttering is placed firmly beyond the pale there is one other possibility to consider. It could well be that the standard methods of establishing whether a person has right or left or incomplete dominance were too unreliable in the past. Certainly it has been found to be most unsatisfactory to try and determine dominance by establishing simply whether the person is right- or left-handed. Even the EEG may be too crude a measuring instrument.

One method that seems to have gone almost unnoticed in this connection has been the phi-test. If there are two bright points of light in a dark room and these are switched on and off alternately, it is possible to see a single point moving from the position of the first to the position of the second. Jasper (1932) used this method for his phi-test and found that the direction in which the light was perceived to move suggested the possible dominant cerebral hemisphere of that person. What was particularly interesting about Jasper's report was that he was able "to classify the stutterers quite definitely with the ambidextrous or left-handed groups of normal speakers". Van Riper (1971) mentions having repeated Jasper's experiment and having obtained the same results.

One other finding that does not quite fit in with the totally negative picture concerning dominance and stuttering is that reported by Jones in

1966. Jones used a test of dominance in which sodium amytal is injected into the carotid artery. If the injection is on the dominant side the cessation of counting lasts several minutes and the counting is confused when it starts again. Jones happened to have four patients who were to be operated on for brain lesions in the temporal region, and who were severe, life-long stutterers. When tested for dominance, these patients were found to respond as if both the right *and* left sides of the brain were dominant. More interesting still, after the operation all four no longer stuttered and all responded to the dominance test on the side that had not been operated on. Jones concluded that "this indicates a transfer of influence to one hemisphere only", and that the results suggested "interference by one hemisphere with the speech performance on the other".

It could just be that the reason why Orton and Travis found no support for their theory was that the method for assessing dominance was not a sufficiently precise one. Although the results of the two studies just mentioned are not enough in themselves to warrant any definite conclusion, interest in the Orton–Travis theory is kept alive. On the other hand, these results do not offer any new support for the supposed association between change of handedness and stuttering. Where this does occur, it could equally well be explained on the grounds of the upset it causes the child; or that parents and other adults who make a child change his preferred hand, and who know of the legendary association with stuttering, will be on the look-out for any signs of incipient stuttering and may convey this anxiety to the child; or that parents who are prepared to correct their child on this issue are of the "correcting" variety and it is this general parental attitude that is at fault.

The Auditory System

There is one rather specialized area of research that has to do with the role of hearing in relation to stuttering. It has been suggested that the stutterer may have some minor disorder of the auditory nervous system. However, several studies have failed to produce any very convincing evidence that this is the case (Gregory, 1964; Shearer and Simmons, 1965).

One particularly interesting aspect of research concerning the relationship between hearing and stuttering has to do with auditory feedback. It has been suggested (Cherry and Sayers, 1956) that stutterers have a defect in the auditory perception of low tones. These authors argue that a person hears his own voice both by the sound travelling through the air *and* through the bones of the skull. When the ears of a stutterer are blocked, so that he receives no air-conducted sound, little change in frequency of stuttering occurs, but when both air- and bone-conducted sounds are eliminated stuttering almost completely disappears.

Cherry and Sayers thought that, since low tones are supposedly conducted through the bone and not the air, cutting out the high frequency tones from the feedback would have little effect on stuttering, while masking the low tone feedback would decrease stuttering. One of the experiments they carried out supported this hypothesis. They stressed however, that their hypothesis was that "stammering is mediated by [note: not *caused* by] the subject's perceptions of his own low-frequency voice sounds . . ."

Several other facts suggest that auditory feedback may play some part in the occurrence of stuttering. The number of stuttering children among the deaf is reported to be only 0.29% to 0.40% (Albright and Malone, 1942), considerably below that found among normal hearing children. Also, if the stutterer is prevented from hearing the sound of his own voice by having a loud noise delivered through earphones while he is speaking, his stuttering is greatly reduced (Maraist and Hutton, 1957; Shane, 1955).

However, Sutton and Chase (1961) argued that being prevented from hearing the *sound* of his own voice may not be the reason for the stutterer's increased fluency since they demonstrated that giving the masking noise in the silent periods *between* speech sounds was equally as effective in reducing stuttering. But Yates (1963) argues that there might still be some auditory masking of speech because normal feedback is not instantaneous. Once again it seems that no definite conclusion can be drawn about the relationship between auditory feedback and stuttering and clearly still more research is needed to clarify the position.

In 1951 Lee wrote a paper entitled "Artificial Stutter". He described how a fluent speaking person could be made to "stutter" by delaying the auditory feedback of the sound of the voice by a short interval. It was not until 1961 that someone decided to try and determine whether, to the listener, the speech disturbance produced in normal speakers by delaying the auditory feedback was of the same kind as that found among stutterers. Neelley (1961) found that the effect on normal speech was definitely not comparable to a stutterer's speech. Seventy-nine per cent of the listeners were able to identify whether a particular sample of speech came from a stutterer or from someone under delayed auditory feedback (DAF). In addition, they were 93% correct in distinguishing between stutterers with and without DAF. Neelley therefore concluded that stuttering and speech behaviour under DAF were quite different and that "an adequate account of stuttering behaviour—or the more comprehensive stuttering problem—is not to be found in the auditory feedback mechanism". However, Yates (1963) argued against accepting these conclusions too readily. He pointed out that Neelley only used one delay interval and that, for normal speakers, reading under DAF is an unusual experience, while reading under ordinary conditions is familiar to stutterers. It is well known that the way in which an individual stutters in adult life is very different from the way in which he stuttered when a child. So perhaps the speech abnormalities produced in people under delayed auditory feedback should be compared with those found in children who stutter rather than with adults. The listener would, however, be able to recognize the different groups by the sound of the voice quite apart from the speech, so a future experiment might compare the difference between the speech of a child with the effect of DAF on the speech of normal speaking children.

An interesting sex difference has been found in the responses to DAF of nonstuttering people. Bachrach (1964) was unable to produce any "artificial stuttering" in eight women but succeeded with eight men, but the two sexes responded to masking tones in the same way. He suggests that these results are consistent with the fact that more men than women stutter.

One possible explanation of these sex differences in response to DAF and masking, and the sex difference found in the incidence of stuttering has been offered by Beech and Fransella (1968). They suggest that, in view of Cherry and Sayers' experimental evidence that stutterers are particularly affected by the perception of low frequency tones, then women will be less likely to stutter, or to "stutter artificially" because their voices "are less likely to be characterized by a preponderance of low frequency tones".

Conclusions

Looking at people who are called stutterers from a physiological, anatomical or neurological standpoint does not enable one to distinguish them from comparable groups of people described as nonstutterers. There have certainly been one or two findings that have not been experimentally contradicted unequivocally but what value are these among so many that have.

The aim in looking for constitutional differences is usually based on some idea of causation. But one is hard put to imagine that a defect as complex as stuttering can be caused by, say, disorders of basal metabolic rate, without this same BMR being sufficiently severe to produce other physiological disorders. It is surely more reasonable to consider that any stutterer/nonstutterer differences in constitution are *the result of* and not the cause of stuttering.

B. PSYCHOLOGICAL CHARACTERISTICS

On the whole, studies into the personality of stutterers have been of two kinds. They have been designed either to find out what particular characteristics stutterers have in common or to find out in what ways stutterers differ from those who do not stutter.

One Group or Many?

Many people have tried very hard to isolate "the stuttering personality" or describe personality traits characteristic of stutterers in general. In this search, one of the common basic assumptions has been that all stutterers can be grouped into a single category—there are not different sorts of stutterers. It becomes a question of great importance whether this assumption holds good when considering the research findings based upon it.

There have been one or two studies that have challenged this assumption. For instance, Douglass and Quarrington (1952) distinguish between "interiorized" and "exteriorized" stutterers. The interiorized stutterer is someone who will go to any length to avoid stuttering, and is sensitive, submissive and retiring. The exteriorized stutterer aims to communicate no matter what happens and will use any avoidance device at his disposal to attain this end; he is aggressive, regards authorities as threatening and never really believes he looks or sounds as abnormal as it can be demonstrated he is.

Quarrington and Douglass (1960) then sub-divided the exteriorized stutterer into "vocalized" and "non-vocalized". The vocalized stutterer is one who can be *heard* to be a stutterer as he repeats syllables and words or prolongs sounds unduly, while the non-vocalized stutterer is one who can be *seen* to be a stutterer by blocking on his words and the curtailment of his speech. These two authors then carried out an experiment to show that the two sub-groups of exteriorized stutterer respond differently to certain situations and so can be regarded as belonging to separate groups. The stutterers were required to read a passage of prose under two conditions. In one case they knew that they could be heard and in the other they were under the impression that they could not. The experimenters predicted, and found, that the non-vocalized stutterer had more reduction in audible stuttering than the vocalized in the situation where he thought he could not be heard, perhaps because he was less anxious about it. How the stutterer views the world affects how he behaves. The authors point out that if there is really a difference between these two sub-groups, then they might well require different types of treatment.

One of the few other studies that have produced results suggesting that sub-groups of stutterers react in different ways to the same situation has been that of Gray and Karmen (1967). They found that severe, mild and moderate stutterers respond differently on measures of anxiety. The moderate stutterer was the odd man out, being more anxious than either the severe or the mild stutterer. This does not necessarily mean that he *felt* more anxious, but just that he was shown to be so on a physiological measure of anxiety in a speaking situation. If anxiety is *not* directly related to severity of stuttering and if people with differing anxiety levels respond differently on some other behavioural measures (e.g. ability to adapt), then researchers using groups of stutterers will have to be very much more rigorous in their selection criteria than they are at present.

The experimental evidence of the existence of qualitatively different sorts of stutterers is by no means conclusive at present, but is compelling enough to make anyone pause and question the assumption that stutterers are sufficiently similar to be studied as if they belong to one group. Maybe it is simply the general ways human beings react to severely incapacitating life-long defects that is being studied.

Research in the behavioural sciences has historically emphasized that science can only be advanced by the study of groups of people, that generalizations cannot be made from data derived from one individual. Critics of this view are becoming more vociferous as people like Baloff and Becker (1967) demonstrate that a curve based on averaged data is dissimilar to the curves of all the individuals whose data contributed to that average. Proponents of single case research such as Shapiro (1961, 1964) argue that research on problems of individuals should be based on the scientific study of the phenomena in these individuals and not on groups. It is conceivable that the stutterers will continue to be sub-divided until research on individuals becomes the order of the day. It is suggested that starting with a theory which focuses upon the individual might lead to more fruitful research than is always the case when one collects basketfuls of facts without theoretical guidance. Bannister and Fransella discuss empirical research thus:

> One of the great illusions in psychology is that 'facts' can be added together and that, come the day of Jubilo, they will be united under one theoretical framework. Only if one works within a theory can an integrated sequence of hypotheses be derived and the experimental findings systematically add to our knowledge. Pure 'fact' gathering is, in any case, a myth. The very selection of this rather than that 'fact' as relevant to our understanding implies assumptions which constitute the psychologist's hidden, unformulated and probably internally contradictory theory. (Bannister and Fransella, 1971, p. 58.)

The Neurotic Stutterer Concept

In the past it was the rule rather than the exception to regard stuttering as a sign of neurosis. The person would not "do" it unless he was basically maladjusted. This attitude, while not all-pervasive, is still to be found among experts (e.g. Barbara, 1958; Sheehan, 1954).

Apart from opinion, what evidence is there that such is the case? In 1942 Bender published the findings of a study under the title "The Stuttering Personality". He had given a test of personality to two hundred and forty-nine male college stutterers and a comparable group of nonstutterers. Beech and Fransella (1968) have criticized the study on statistical grounds, but point out that the results do suggest that the stuttering American college students investigated were more introverted, less dominant, less confident and less sociable than the nonstuttering students. But this can just as likely be the *effect* of stuttering as its cause.

Bender's study proved to be the incentive for a whole spate of attempts to show that the stutterer possesses certain characteristic personality traits including his being more "neurotic" than others. Walnut (1954), for example, gave the Minnesota Multiphasic Personality Inventory (MMPI) to a control group, a group of stutterers, a group of cripples and a group of people with cleft palates. He found no abnormal features of personality in any of the groups. All the scores fell below the 70th rank (the level suggested by the MMPI manual at which an item should be considered clinically significant). However, Walnut comments on significant differences on certain items between the control and the "pathological" group. He says "The stuttering group showed significant differences on the Depression and Paranoid scales and these differences were toward the poor adjustment end of the scale". According to the MMPI manual this would indicate that, in relation to others of comparable experience, the stuttering group has (1) "poor adjustment of the emotional type with a feeling of uselessness and inability to assume normal optimism with regard to the future", and is characterized by (2) "suspiciousness, over sensitivity, and delusions of persecution". In fact, all that was really being compared were differences in degree of *normality* and not the presence or absence of *abnormal* features.

The caution with which one must approach interpretations of results has been stressed by many writers. In particular, Sheehan (1958) points out that in one study (Krugman, 1946) the interpretation of results was that child stutterers have an "obsessive-compulsive" type of personality, whereas the statistical analysis of the results had been a direct contradiction of this interpretation. Although the psychoanalysts commonly associate stuttering and obsessional character traits, this has proved hard to support experimentally (Bloodstein and Schreiber, 1957).

If one were forced to reach a conclusion about whether or not stutterers as a group are more neurotic than nonstutterers then, on the basis of positive evidence, one would have to bring in the verdict of *not proven*.

This is because so many of the studies have employed faulty statistics or unsound reasoning, have lacked proper controls or the authors have misinterpreted or over-extended the interpretation of their results.

Luckily however, one does not have to reach a conclusion on only these rather shaky positive findings. The negative findings far outweigh them. Studies reporting no evidence of neurotic tendencies in the stutterer groups are not all free from the criticisms levelled against the studies producing positive findings. But taking the mass of evidence that exists, there is nothing to suggest that the stutterer is any more or less likely to be neurotic than the next man, and the person who insists that there is, will find little hard fact to back up his contention.

One point that has tended to be overlooked in many of these studies is that most of the samples of stutterers have included far more men than women. When separate analyses of the response of men and women have been carried out, considerable sex differences have been found. For instance, Madison and Norman (1952) found female but not male stutterers to have higher than normal "Need-Persistence" and males but not females to be less "Extrapunitive". Walnut (1954) found that his female stutterers differed significantly (but within the normal range) from the male stutterers on one of the scales on the MMPI. Anastasi (1958) has stressed that in general women tend to get more neurotic or maladjusted scores than men on personality tests. On the basis of this one could argue that, when investigators use the data published with the test against which to compare their stutterers' responses, they may be loading the dice in favour of getting negative results. However, although this may be a factor in the failure to demonstrate the existence of the "neurotic stutterer", it seems highly unlikely that it is powerful enough to submerge him if he really existed in large numbers.

The Stutterer's Personality Characteristics

Similarly conflicting results have been characteristic of studies that have tried to find particular clusters of personality traits that might characterize the stutterer. One cannot help but be struck again by the great weight of negative findings in this search, and how it seems easier to find ways in which the stutterer does *not* differ from the nonstutterer than ways in which he does. If there really were a general personality profile possessed by the majority of stutterers one would have expected something concrete to have emerged by this time from the large amount of research that has been conducted.

Apart from interest in trying to identify the general personality profile of the stutterer there has, in recent years, been some research into more specific personality variables.

3

Level of Aspiration. One such variable is that of "level of aspiration". In a typical situation the subject takes a shot at a target and makes a score. He is told his score and asked what score he expects to make on the next shot. A measure of the difference between his expectation and his achievement is then obtained. On the whole, stutterers tend to underestimate the score they will get on the next trial, but whether this is so for other groups with long-standing defects is not known. Sex differences have again been found (Sheehan and Zelen, 1955), the female stutterers getting lower scores but having less discrepancy between their aim and achievement than the males. The authors point out that this is interesting in view of the still mysterious sex ratio differences in stuttering. They express the hope that a full-scale investigation of such differences will soon be forthcoming; but seventeen years later this hope has yet to be fulfilled.

Anxiety. Not only have most people been of the opinion that severity of stuttering is related to the level of anxiety in that person at a particular time, but some think that the stutterer is generally more anxious than the nonstutterer. Johnson and Spielberger (1968) refer to these two aspects as "state" and "trait" anxiety; the former being a reaction to the stress of the moment and the latter being an enduring feature of the personality.

Santostefano (1960) thinks that the stutterer is under constant stress because of the poor opinion he has of himself and he thinks others have of him. He feels that this produces 'predominant and enduring states of anxiety and hostility'. In support of these ideas about "trait" anxiety, he reports finding that a group of stutterers had higher anxiety and hostility scores on the Rorschach Inkblot Test than did nonstutterers. Although he administered the fifty-two Rorschachs himself, the protocols were coded so that he scored them one week later with no knowledge of whether they belonged to a stutterer or not. He also demonstrated that the stutterers were less able to perform well on a laboratory task when they were put under stress—they were less able to recall emotionally-arousing words that they had previously learned (see also Adams, 1969). But apart from this study there is little to support the idea that stutterers are generally more anxious than nonstutterers.

Gray and Karmen (1967), however, report no difference in anxiety level between stutterers and nonstutterers in the laboratory situation when the measure is a physiological one. But when the stutterers were divided up in terms of severity of speech defect, the moderate stutterers had a higher level of anxiety than did the others. It could be that most of Santostefano's stutterers were of the "moderate" type, but this seems unlikely.

Nearly every account of stuttering implies a relationship between anxiety and the disfluent act but, as Ingham and Andrews (1972a) point out, there is little or no evidence for this belief. Treatment procedures, such as systematic desensitization, are based on the assumption that if the anxiety reaction to specific situations is reduced, a reduction in stuttering will occur. Ingham and Andrews measured "state" anxiety on the basis of responses to a questionnaire in eight stutterers under treatment. They found that, although the number of disfluencies was reduced substantially, the amount of expressed anxiety remained high. While this finding provides no definitive answer it does raise the question of whether such a direct link between anxiety and severity of stuttering exists as is so often assumed.

Self Concepts. Recent interest has focused on the self concept of stutterers, defined as "the self as the individual is known to himself" (English and English, 1958). There are several "self concept" theories, most of whose authors speculate about the "self we know ourselves to be" as opposed to "our environment" and reflect that the relationship between these two determines behaviour. Others, such as Kelly (1955), see the notion of the self as being related to other ways in which individuals view their world. Each man sees himself in relation to those ideas he uses to construe others. He may see himself as weak, kind and generous in relation to his wife and firm, stern and cautious in relation to his employees.

Within the field of stuttering, many authorities have emphasized the importance of the notion of the stutterer's "self-concept" and its relation to treatment. Shearer (1961) sees much of a treatment programme being "devoted to reconciling the two conflicting self-concepts, the horrible stuttering self and the free speaking normal self" and suggests that the stutterer relapses if he ceases to perceive himself as someone who stutters. Sheehan (1954) also talks of a dichotomized self-concept. He comments that the thought of suddenly ceasing to stutter often produces anxiety "Because the defect may become a peg on which to hang all his shortcomings . . . He may have lived with his stuttering so long that functioning without it involved too radical a change in self-concept to be readily assimilated." He goes on to say that 'Just as in the early stages of treatment, the stutterer needs to accept himself as a stutterer, so in the final stages he must learn to accept himself as a normal speaker. The second adjustment is sometimes bigger than the first'.

Various methods of measurement have been used to examine whether the self-concept of the stutterer differs from that of the nonstutterer. Wallen (1959) succeeded in differentiating the two groups by showing stutterers to be less independent, more lacking in emotional control, less self-accepting and more self-rejecting. The stutterer group also had a greater discrepancy between how each individual saw himself as he was and how he would like to be. Using another method of measurement, Fiedler and Wepman (1951) failed to find any differences. Part of the difficulties encountered in such studies seems to be lack of a clear idea about what the self-concept is and, thus, what is actually being measured.

Instead of comparing the self-concept of stutterers with that of non-stutterers, Fransella (1968) tried to establish whether the stutterer sees himself as "a stutterer". She used two measuring methods, one of them (a special form of the semantic differential [Smith, 1962; Fransella, 1965a, b]) was given to nonstutterers as well. All ratings on a set of nine semantic differential scales were subjected to factor analysis, and Fig. 1

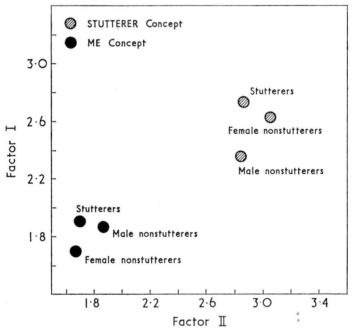

Fig. 1. Concepts *Me* and *Stutterers* used by stutterers, male and female nonstutterers on a semantic differential plotted along the first two factors (Fransella, 1968).

shows two concepts—*me* and *stutterers*—plotted along the two main dimensions of meaning. The chance that these differences in meaning occurred by chance alone is less than one in a hundred. The stutterers did not associate the idea of themselves with the idea of being a stutterer. The unexpected finding was that the stutterers (all males) and both sexes of nonstutterers do not differ significantly in the way they rated those concepts. Perhaps this is a stereotyped view of the stutterer which the stutterer himself also holds. On the face of it, he holds himself aloof from the group to which, by definition, he belongs. He is unique. He stutters but in no other respect is he like the rest of the group he calls stutterers.

Stereotypes, like rules are perhaps made to be broken. A moment's reflection is all that is needed to remind us that as soon as we get to know

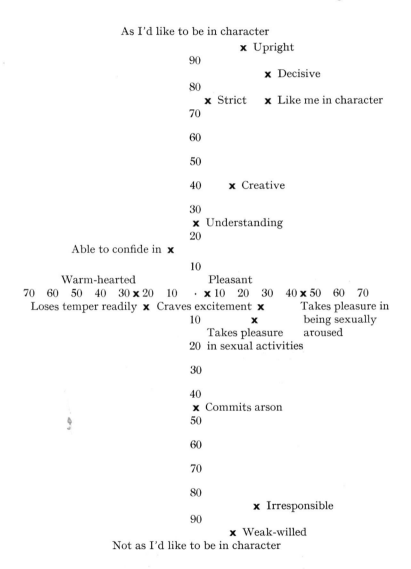

FIG. 2. Constructs used by an arsonist plotted along the two main dimensions of his repertory grid (Fransella and Adams, 1966).

someone, that person is often made the exception to the general rule that had previously embraced him. Just so the stutterer makes an exception of himself.

It seems possible that the stutterer is not the only person who refuses to be categorized as "people" say he should. A similar effect was found in another study (Fransella and Adams, 1966). In Fig. 2 it is clear that, while the "self" is associated with *uprightness* and the *"ideal" self*, people who commit arson are *irresponsible, weak-willed* and *not as he would like to be*. This man was, in fact, a person society called an arsonist. He was serving a prison sentence for this offence. Yet, quite clearly he was not "that sort of person" in his own eyes, just as the stutterer is not like other stutterers in his own terms. A similar effect has been shown with alcoholics (Hoy, 1972).

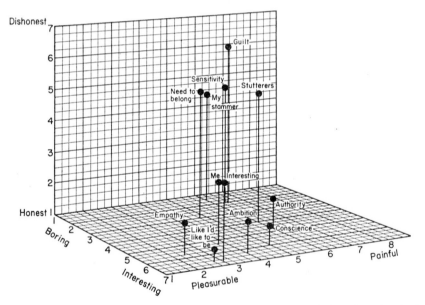

FIG. 3. Concepts used by a stutterer on a semantic differential plotted along the first three factors (Fransella, 1965a).

One explanation of this might be sought in the notion of stereotypes. For the arsonist, people who commit arson are evaluatively *"bad"*. Figure 3 is a plot of the self and "stutterer" concepts along three dimensions of meaning for an individual stutterer. This, in fact, was the general pattern for all, with the concept *me* being seen as "Interesting", slightly "Pleasurable", and "Honest" rather than "Dishonest", and *stutterers* as "Painful" and "Dishonest" but neither "Interesting" nor "Boring".

Conlon (1966) asked nonstuttering college students to rate themselves once as they are and once as if they were stutterers. They likewise evaluated themselves in positive and 'stutterers' in negative terms. Most people will not readily see themselves in such a bad light and stutterers are no exception.

Shearer (1961) talks about the horrible stuttering self and the free-speaking self and says that this is the dual self-concept. But perhaps that statement should be altered to say that there is the "speaker-who-stutters self" and the "person-that-has-nothing-to-do-with-speaking self". If there is a different set of concepts to describe each "self", then there should be no conflict of the sort Shearer suggests. The stutter is viewed as being like measles, something imposed from outside.

The reason why some people have obtained results indicating that the stutterer *does* see himself as one is that if he is asked he will obviously say he is. But using more indirect techniques, one can establish that many see themselves in as individual terms as anyone else—they are only stutterers when speaking.

Conclusions

It is often thought that stereotypes are based on some observation which, as a generalization, holds good. If this is so, then some psychological or physiological factor other than the stutter should be observable and should make stutterers identifiable as a group. However, having looked at a sample of the studies attempting to identify such common factors, the conclusion must be that there is no evidence that the stutterer differs from the nonstutterer in any clearly identifiable way, other than by his speech.

However, it must be remembered that this is a statement about a group and not about individuals. It simply means that, taking a group of stutterers at random and a comparable group of nonstutterers, one would find quiet and talkative ones, aggressive and meek ones, intelligent and stupid ones *in each group. From the knowledge that a person is a stutterer one can predict little about him, except that he will more probably be a man than a woman, is liable to be 'thrown' by situations he perceives as stressful and undervalues his future performance.* If there are as many sub-groups of stutterers as there are sub-groups of men, what price stuttering research? Perhaps one should concentrate solely on the behaviour of stuttering rather than the stutterer. Alternatively, perhaps there is something in the way in which he views the world that makes him perpetuate the behaviour in spite of the discomfort it causes him; perhaps it is better than being precipitated into a world of which he has only limited direct knowledge.

CHAPTER 2

The Treatment of Stuttering Down the Ages

I slaved my life out over breathing, vocal and articulatory exercises by the aid
of books; but, however much I pondered over the cause of the suffering and
watched its different symptoms, all my pains proved futile, nor was I spared the
disheartening realization that those fetters did but strengthen the more I
worked to rid myself of them. Eventually I decided to place myself under the
care of specialists who professed to be able to eradicate the affliction. I visited
institutes for the cure of stammering—as many as three !—all in vain, however.
I am confident that I did my utmost to carry out all instructions with the
greatest conscientiousness and perseverance . . . I came to the conclusion that
by far the largest percentage (*at least* 90 per cent.) of those who have been
discharged as 'cured' are, in reality, only seemingly cured, and, when my
investigations led me to discover that dread of speaking and inner psychic
resistances are the cause of the complaint, I knew that mechanical exercises
would not remove such subtle difficulties, and that a real and lasting cure was
yet to be found.

The Real Cause of Stammering and its Permanent Cure
Alfred Appelt (1911)

I. Theory and Treatment

The speech disorder that today we call stuttering has had quite a
chequered career. It may well be as old as speech itself, but whether it
took the same form as today is beyond our capacity to determine. Certainly some of the speech defects of "famous" stutterers are rather poorly
described. For instance, Moses is recorded in most writings as having been
a stutterer. Yet, can we really be sure exactly what his speech defect was?

And Moses said unto the Lord, O my Lord, I am not eloquent neither hereto-
fore, nor since has thou spoken unto thy servant; but I am slow of speech,
and of a slow tongue. (Exod. IV, 10.)

Whether one defines Moses' slowness of speech as stuttering or not, the
prognosis for some was good.

Isaiah says:

And the eyes of them that see shall not be dim, and the ears of them that
hear shall harken.
 The heart also of the rash shall understand knowledge, and the tongue of
the stammerers shall be ready to speak plainly. (Isa. XXXII, 3–4.)

The diagnostic confusion over speech impediments is common in early
writings as, for instance, over the difference between stuttering and
lisping. It is possible that Demosthenes was more a lisper, unable to

articulate the letter, than a stutterer. Eldridge (1968) speaks of Demosthenes' "lisping, breathless, hesitant speech", and of how his first speaking appearance in public life was an appalling fiasco:

> The moment he began to speak, his fate was sealed. His weak, breathless voice and his lisping utterance and, worst of all, his hesitance, were too much for his critical audiences. He was greeted with shouts of laughter. (Eldridge, 1968, p. 12.)

The idea that stuttering is not only a physical affliction but is also genetically determined, persists today both in scientific and lay thinking. Somerset Maugham, for instance, remarks that:

> We're the product of our genes and chromosomes. And there's nothing whatever we can do about it . . . no one can. Because we can't change the essential natures we're born with . . . All we can do is to try and supplement our own deficiencies. (French, 1966.)

One of the snags about a theory of a constitutional basis of stuttering is that it fosters the attitude that, as Maugham says, there is nothing whatever one can do about it. However, if we take the position that the only thing that is constitutionally determined is a poorer than average verbal ability, and that the environment does the rest, then clearly there should be something one can do. Not all children who have difficulty in learning to speak become stutterers.

The theory that one holds about a disorder or a piece of behaviour determines what one does about changing that form of behaviour. Those holding an "all-or-none" genetic theory will try and teach stutterers to "supplement their own deficiencies"; the learning theorist may aim to reciprocally inhibit the undesired response or manipulate its contingencies, and the psychodynamic theorist search for psychic conflicts.

The case for using theory in approaching treatment has been strongly put by Erasmus Darwin, and he links theory with therapy as follows:

> 1. *Titubatie linguae.* Impediment of speech is owing to the associations of the motions of the organs of speech being interrupted or dissevered by ill-employed sensations or sensitive motions, as by awe, bashfulness, ambition of shining, or fear of not succeeding, and the person uses voluntary efforts in vain to regain the broken associations . . .
>
> The broken association is generally between the fifth consonant and the succeeding vowel; as in endeavouring to pronounce the word parable, the p is voluntarily repeated again and again, but the remainder of the word does not follow, because the association between it and the next vowel is dissevered.
>
> The art of curing this defect is to cause the stammerer to repeat the word, which he finds difficult to speak, eight or ten times without the initial letter, in a strong voice, or with an aspirate before it, as arable or harable; and at length to speak it very softly with the initial letter p, parable. This should be practiced for weeks or months upon every word, which the stammerer hesitates

in pronouncing. To this should be added much commerce with mankind, in order to acquire a carelessness about the opinions of others. (Darwin, 1801, Vol. 4, p. 289.)

This form of therapy would certainly not be considered unusual today, but Bacon's theory might, because it has particularly pleasant therapeutic implications:

Divers, we See, doe Stut. The Cause may be, (in most) the Refrigeration of the Tongue; Whereby it is lesse apt to move. And therefore we See, that Naturalls doe generally Stut: And we see, that those that Stut, if they drink Wine moderately, they Stut lesse, because it heateth: And so we See, that they that Stut, doe Stut more in the first offer to speake, than in Continuance; Because the Tongue is, by Motion, somewhat heateth. In some also it may be, (though rarely) the Drinesse of the Tongue; which like-wise maketh it lesse apt to move, as well as Cold; for it is an Affect that commeth to some Wise and Great Men; As it did unto Moses who was Lingua praepedita; and many Stutters (we finde) are very Cholericke Men; Choler Enducing a Drinesse in the Tongue. (Bacon, 1627, p. 101).

II. Treatment Past and Present

A. THE PHYSICAL APPROACH

Apart from the writings of Darwin and Bacon, stuttering was discussed much earlier by many people including Hippocrates, Aristotle, and Galen (Bluemel, 1957). Hippocrates thought that the stammerer was full of black bile and preceded Bacon in thinking that it resulted from loss of heat. While Aristotle wrote that:

When people stammer, it is due, not to an affection of the veins but to the movement of the tongue; for they find a difficulty in changing the position of the tongue when they have to utter a second sound. (Forster, 1927.)

In the 14th century there was a change from mechanical theories emphasizing the tongue as the cause of stuttering to physiological theories of causation. Guy de Chauliac, for instance, considered stuttering to result from ulcers of the tongue and advocated treatment by the "application of embrocations, cauteries, blisters and gargles for the tongue" (Eldridge, 1968).

Right up to the 19th century explanations as to the cause of stuttering were, in general, centred upon some idea of the malfunctioning of the tongue. Unsoundness of speech muscles, weakness of the soft palate and uvula, faulty positioning of the tongue, too short a tongue. All and many others were cited as causes.

No treatment is ever carried out without the therapist having some theory about causation, although often only implicitly. This is perhaps particularly so when considering the spate of anatomical explanations and surgical remedies of the 19th century. Dieffenbach (1841) wrote about a new surgical operation to cure stuttering by cutting a transverse wedge out of the tongue and then sewing the raw edges together, and many surgeons followed him with refinements of their own. Others used less drastic methods, being largely content to cut the frenum of the tongue, or pierce the tongue with hot needles. All these methods of cure arose from the theory that the stutterer's tongue was set incorrectly in the mouth.

Later, causation was thought to result from faulty respiration and speech musculature, resulting in breathing and speech exercises. Bluemel is of the opinion that Canon Kingsley had a great influence on the pattern of British speech therapy, believing as he did that breath control was central to the problem and had as his formula 'take full breaths and plenty of them'. Yet Bluemel points out that this idea may well have gone back more than two thousand years to the time when Satyrus made Demosthenes do speech exercises while walking—he had to stride along the beach and shout to make himself heard above the sea.

Present day techniques are varied indeed, many of them stemming directly from centuries' old beliefs.

Relaxation

Techniques of relaxation were introduced formally into therapy in England before the end of the last century and still hold an important place today. Bluemel reports Hoffman as saying in 1840 that "the utmost relaxation of the body must prevail during speech". Similarly, in 1967 Brutten and Shoemaker state that:

> This therapeutic strategy (relaxation) derives from the assumption that as the stutterer becomes increasingly relaxed he will become less fearful of the clinical setting and more capable of considering the emotional stimuli. (Brutten and Shoemaker, 1967, p. 101.)

Rhythm

Another therapeutic procedure with a venerable history is the use of rhythm. This comes from the common observation that the stutterer very often does not stutter when he speaks rhythmically. When recommending the use of the "rhythmus of Milton" in 1810, Thelwell observed:

> But how little the real sources of impediment are in general understood, will be obvious to those who have had the opportunity of observing that even those very impediments, so merely and exclusively vocal, are seldom, if ever, found to affect the voice in singing.

Although Thelwell claims not to have understood the defect very well, he clearly thought it to be of articulatory rather than of, say, psychological origin. It was Colombat de l'Isere (1840) who popularized the use of speaking in single syllables in rhythm, accompanied by placing the thumb and forefinger together. Later he constructed an instrument for the purpose, the "Muthonome", which eventually was sold commercially as the metronome.

The use of rhythm as a therapeutic aid is still with us in the present day. In 1940 Van Dantzig reports the use of regularly stressed syllables either by itself or as part of the treatment programme. The presence of rhythm has not always been made explicit as in the case of Kastein (1947) who used "chewing therapy"; but if you chew while you talk, you talk in a slow syllabic monotone.

Meyer and Mair (1963) studied five stutterers and their response to treatment based on artificially imposed rhythmic speech. Meyer then devised an ingenious hearing-aid through which rhythmic sounds were transmitted. Like an ordinary hearing-aid, it was possible to turn the "beats" on and off. Thus, in the first instance the stutterer was instructed to turn the device on whenever he wanted to say something. Next he switched it off but spoke "as if" it were still present. Finally, he dispensed with it altogether. Some of the stutterers showed initial improvement with this, but there was a tendency to relapse. Meyer and Comley (1967) followed up this pilot study with the treatment of a group of forty-eight stutterers. The group used the hearing aid outside the clinical situation in an attempt to encourage the generalization of rhythmic speech to the social environment. Each stutterer was instructed to use the rhythmic aid first in the least stressful conditions and then in progressively more difficult ones. A control group was instructed in rhythmic speech in the same way, but had no artificial aid.

Of their reported sample of forty-eight stutterers, seventeen were unable to master rhythmic speech and showed no significant speech improvement at the end of treatment. An analysis of these rhythmic non-responders showed the majority to have their speech characterized by "hard blocking" and were judged the least fluent. The remaining members of both experimental and control groups improved significantly and had retained the improvement twenty-four weeks after treatment had stopped. There here seems some evidence of a treatment that is comparatively short (maximum of sixteen sessions), and which is effective for stutterers rated as moderate and who are able to impose a rhythmicity into their speech at an initial test session. However, final evaluation must await the full report of these results.

Brady (1968) reports a treatment programme in which a similar battery-operated metronome designed as a hearing aid was used with six stutterers in conjunction with psychotherapy. "The acquisition of greater fluency may mean the loss of secondary gains which have accrued to the speech disorder. Problems of these kinds often require skilful psychotherapeutic handling". At the time of the report three of the stutterers have "acquired fluency within the normal limit", but no details are provided. In subsequent work he used the metronome in conjunction with a programme of systematic desensitization (see p. 37).

As with nearly all treatments based upon manipulation of the speech, many other factors are involved. For instance, in Brady's study "treatment sessions are spent mainly in attempting to help patients deal with their own specific difficulties, utilizing relaxation and—where necessary and possible—simulated social situations". Therefore, the evaluation of the effect of rhythm as a treatment technique is difficult.

Andrews and Harris (1964) report the use of syllable-timed speech as a therapeutic measure. In this the stutterer is "taught to speak syllable by syllable, stressing each syllable evenly saying each in time to a regular even rhythm". They report that all their subjects responded well to this artificial speech for at least a few days but that relapse occurred to some extent in most of them. In a more recent study, Brandon and Harris (1967) gave extensive treatment of this type to ten stutterers. These were treated as in-patients for the first week and as day patients for the second week. The next eighteen stutterers were given two weeks' treatment as day attenders. Of the total twenty-eight stutterers, eighteen, or 64%, improved by a reduction of speech errors of 60% or more. It is difficult to tell from the report whether this is the figure after eighteen months follow-up or immediately after the end of treatment. If it is after eighteen months follow-up then it is a procedure with definite merit. However, the treatment involved other procedures besides syllable-timed speech. For instance, when discussing the change of programme for the second group the authors state that "other changes have involved actual reinforcement programmes for the evening sessions, where syllable timing is practised continuously, and more discussion of difficulties arising as a result of increased fluency".

Recently, Ingham and Andrews (1972b) reported the results of a comparison of the effectiveness of four treatment techniques which included the use of syllable-timed speech. They found that this significantly reduced the frequency of stuttering but that, when it was used in treatment in conjunction with a "token reinforcement system", both frequency of stuttering and rate of speech approached that of nonstutterers. These results were based on fifty-eight stutterers who received treatment during a twelve-day (100-hour) intensive course. Whether the improvement reported was maintained at the nine-month follow-up has yet to be reported.

Shadowing

Another type of treatment related to the use of rhythm is based on perceptual rather than motor functions. Cherry and Sayers (1956) hypothesize that ". . . stammering (functionally) represents a type of relaxation oscillation, caused by instability of the feedback loop". They relate this to all the studies testing the idea that the rhythm effect is the result of distraction or taking the stutterer's attention away from the sound of his own voice. They mention the report of Kern (1932) whose stutterers read fluently while being partially deafened by the sound of a drum.

Cherry and Sayers discuss their hypothesis (they are careful to point out that they do not think of it as a formal theory) in relation to the technique of "shadowing". In this, the stutterer "shadows" the words uttered by a second speaker reading from a book. The stutterer is thus concentrating very hard on the reader and so has little time to perceive his own utterances. They used this speech-shadowing technique as a form of treatment for children and adults, but assessment as to the efficacy of this method is not possible as only case study reports are available.

However, Krikler (personal communication) gave fifty stutterers experience in shadowing for a period of eight weeks and found a high percentage of initial improvement, but this was not maintained in those who did not receive additional psychotherapy or more general behavioural treatment. A few who did receive the additional treatment had maintained improvement at follow-up. She found no relationship between degree of improvement and initial severity. Kŏndas (1969) also used the procedure with children, together with breathing exercises, and reported that 70% have been successfully treated, but once again the results cannot be assessed as no details are given.

Drugs

An implicit belief that stuttering has an organic or neurological basis is evident in those who today attempt to treat stuttering by the use of drugs. But the majority of results have not been encouraging. One of the first studies (Love, 1955) involved each stutterer reading different passages of prose having had either a depressant, a stimulant, a placebo or no drug at all. No difference was found in the number of speech errors produced.

However, drug studies have been reported where tranquillizers have been given as a therapeutic tool. Mitchell (1955) used reserpine which produced a general improvement in attitude and in amount of subjective anxiety reported by the stutterers, but there was no significant improvement in speech fluency. Chlorpromizine has also been used (e.g. Hackett *et al.*, 1958; Winkelman, 1954), this time with more encouraging results. But against this one must set the evidence of Heaver *et al.* (cited by Kent, 1963) who used reserpine and chlorpromizine in a controlled study and reported that the drug groups could not be differentiated from the placebo groups. Kent also reports that Winkelman told her that his ratings of improvement were based on subjective observations and that no objective ratings of anxiety or speech were attempted. Meprobamate has met with no greater measure of success.

Thus, while there is some evidence that tranquillizer drugs serve to reduce anxiety and tension, they still have to be shown to have a significant effect on stuttering itself. Added to this lack of convincing evidence of the effectiveness of the drugs as a therapeutic device must be the fact that several of the research studies report having used some form of speech therapy or psychotherapy as well.

Recently, Wells and Malcolm (1971) used the drug haloperidol in a controlled study with and without speech therapy. They found that the drug did produce significant improvement in their group of thirty-six stutterers and they "formed the impression that improvement continued at least for some weeks after stopping treatment". This result suggests the need for further research to determine, among other things, whether the drug is entirely responsible for the improvement or merely provides the right psychological climate for some rethinking on the part of the stutterer to take place.

Shock

Following up the belief that the stutterer has some neurological or biochemical malfunctioning of the brain, Owen and Stemmermann (1947) administered electroconvulsive therapy to stutterers and reported good results. To the author's knowledge, no one has replicated this study and it is difficult to see why they should except under the theoretical head "anything is worth a try".

Conclusions

Up to the present day, many methods of physical treatment have not changed greatly since the defect was first being discussed. In the few instances in which research has been carried out, the lack of detailed data make the results extremely difficult to assess. In addition to this, therapies using manipulation of speech, drugs and so forth, very often incorporate some psychological therapy as well. While there are still people who believe that stuttering has some physical cause then physical treatments will persist. The onus is on them to show that the results obtained by their method are achieved *independently* of any psychological change or at least to show what the relationship between the two factors is.

Ideas to do with the psychological make-up of the stutterer can also be traced back to the dim and distant past, but these have only been made explicit in the last hundred years or so.

In 1844 Klencke states that stuttering is

> The outcome of a want of freedom of the soul with regard to the stimuli of that most important part of culture, speech.

This "want of freedom of the soul" is, for him, the result of insufficient co-ordination of the spinal chord and of the brain. But he emphasized that the whole person should be treated and not just the speech.

Thomé (1867) took this one step further by placing the basic cause of stuttering on an abnormality of the central nervous system, but at the same time believing that this malfunctioning was psychologically induced. It could be produced by such things as embarrassment and lack of confidence, also by excessively rapid thought which was in turn accompanied by an effort to produce speech with corresponding rapidity.

This line of thought led to the theory that stuttering was of psycho-neurotic origin (Ssikorski, 1894). But still there was the proviso that this psychoneurosis had neurological foundations and that it was the *precipitation* of stuttering that was evoked by psychic stimuli.

Treatments based on the idea that there is some important psychological component that causes the stutterer to stutter are perhaps not as bizarre as some of the physical treatments, but they are certainly varied.

Psychotherapy

Notions concerning the psychoneurotic base of stuttering are still widely held today and the lack of experimental evidence to back them up has been discussed. From a position that says "stutterers are neurotic" the obvious step to take is to treat the speech defect by some form of psychotherapy. Little or no attention is paid to the speech act itself; concentration is on the person. One of the earliest exponents of this approach was Appelt (1911). He was convinced that

> An essential of successful treatment is the clear realization of the manner in which the stammerer has built round himself a complicated system of psychic reactions which is intended to protect him.

He sees the therapist's task as one in which he has to get full insight into the stutterer's mental life so that he can substitute more appropriate qualities for the "neurotic" qualities the stutterer possesses.

The most commonly used form of non-symptomatic psychotherapy is dynamic in orientation (e.g. Barbara, 1958). One of the few deviators from this path is Hejna (1960), who reports a treatment programme based on Rogers' Client-centred Therapy (1961). At the present point in time it is impossible to evaluate the success of these non-symptomatic psychotherapeutic approaches in reducing or eliminating stuttering, since no systematic research has been reported in any detail.

Behaviour Therapy

By far the most notable addition to the theoretical explanations of stuttering has been to regard it as learned behaviour—having been learned then it might be unlearned. This is not necessarily so, of course; no law operates which says that what goes in *has* to come out. There are a number of theories that view stuttering as some form of conditioned or learned behaviour and a rapidly increasing volume of research reports indicate the possible usefulness of this view.

Systematic Desensitization. Two main approaches currently designed to eliminate the undesired behaviour using a learning theory model are the desensitization and operant procedures. In the former, the aim is to replace the anxiety produced by certain stimuli with a response that is incompatible with anxiety. Wolpe (1958) considers that anxiety is at the core of nearly all neuroses and that "speaking to people without stuttering is made possible for these subjects by eliminating their neurotic anxiety habit of response to people" (Wolpe, 1969). One way Wolpe believes a person can be helped to exchange anxiety for another type of reaction is to teach him to relax and then get him to imagine the previously anxiety-provoking situations. Alternatively, the person can be made to actually encounter the situations that normally produce anxiety. He is introduced to them gradually, while pleasant company and the discussion of topics of interest lead him to experience a general feeling of well-being in the previously anxiety-provoking situations. The relaxation method has the advantage over the method using real-life situations as it can take place within the consulting room.

Both desensitization procedures involve the establishing of a hierarchy of situations that are presumed to produce different levels of anxiety, extending from those eliciting almost no anxiety to those eliciting maximum anxiety. These hierarchies are usually derived by taking a very detailed account from the individual of the situations relating to the undesired behaviour. Considerable experience is needed to make sure that the situations in the hierarchy are not graded in such a way that the jump in anxiety-provoking potential is too great between any of the steps. A method for establishing the degree to which one step differs from another in numerical terms is given in Chapter 8.

4

If, as many believe, stuttering is closely related to anxiety, then removal of the anxiety should produce a decrease in stuttering. Gray and Karmen (1967) however, found that this may not be so for all stutterers. They suggest that desensitization may be effective with moderately severe stutterers who have a high level of anxiety but not so effective with mild or severe stutterers, both of whom they found to have low levels of anxiety.

There have been two research reports of the use of systematic desensitization with stutterers. Lanyon (1969) treated one man whose stuttering was assessed as "slightly less than average" in severity. The feared situations were presented to him while he was in a state of deep relaxation. At the end of sixteen sessions the young man was reported to have improved 56% on a measure of speaking and 40% on a measure of reading. At a nine-month follow-up there was further improvement. Lanyon points out that no generalizations can be made from this one study but suggests that further research could profitably be carried out into the usefulness of this method.

In a more extensive piece of research, Brady (1971) combined the use of rhythm with desensitization. Twenty-six adult stutterers were first taught to pace their speech to the beat of a metronome, both while alone and in the presence of someone with whom stuttering was at a minimum. The desk metronome was then replaced by a miniaturized version, which can be worn unobtrusively. A hierarchy of situations was then constructed from most to least likely to produce stuttering. The stutterers used the metronome to practice speaking in each of these situations in order of increasing difficulty. They then repeated speaking in this same hierarchy of situations without the metronome. Brady reports that "90% showed a marked increase in fluency" and that this had persisted over the follow-up periods to date. Perhaps even more striking than this very high level of improvement is that the average number of treatment sessions was only 11·8. Again, unfortunately, no more detailed figures are given.

Operant Conditioning. As with desensitization, operant approaches to the elimination of stuttering have been more argued and speculated about than investigated experimentally. In this approach, the behaviour is not considered to be dependent upon the presence of anxiety. It is considered to be maintained by the consequences of stuttering. Goldiamond (1969) points out that stuttering can produce "punishment" by the listener and so, if there is any anxiety, it is the *result of* rather than the cause of stuttering. Goldiamond emphasizes that the operant approach concentrates on behaviour that succeeds (fluency) and not on that which fails (stuttering).

One of the earlier reports on the effect of using the consequences of disfluency as the source of control, was that of Flanagan *et al.* (1958). In their experiment, stutterers in one situation were given a loud noise through ear-phones immediately they stuttered; in the other the stutterers could "escape" a continual noise *by stuttering*. The authors concluded that by showing stuttering to decrease when it was followed by an unpleasant consequence and to increase when it *enabled* the stutterer to escape from a continuous unpleasant situation, they had demonstrated that stuttering is affected by its consequences. However, Biggs and Sheehan (1969) repeated this experiment, with certain modifications, and found stuttering to decrease when it was followed by punishment and to decrease also when the stuttering caused a continuous unpleasant noise to cease. They concluded that the noise serves only as a distraction device.

Whether this is so or not does not alter the fact that there is impressive evidence that speech disfluencies in the stutterer *and* in the normal speaker can be modified by their consequences (e.g. Siegel and Martin, 1965 a, b; Goldiamond, 1965) *in the laboratory situation*.

When the operant approach is applied to the permanent elimination of stuttering, one of the main problems is to identify the consequence that leads to its continuation. If the consequences of stuttering were punishing, it should, logically, be eliminated. But it is not. Therefore, say the operant theorists, there must be some other consequence that is rewarding. Goldiamond (1969) cites the apparently masochistic pigeon which pecked at a disc even though it got an unpleasant shock each time (Holz and Azrin, 1961). When the shock was turned off, pecking soon ceased. However, the pigeon was getting food at every fiftieth peck when the shock was on, and a second experiment showed that the trained pigeon would peck at a disc to get food at every fiftieth peck even without shock. It was this infrequent supply of food that seemed to be producing the "masochistic" behaviour.

Goldiamond thus emphasizes the importance of finding out what the consequence is that is maintaining the stuttering. If this is not done, the stuttering may be removed but some other undesired behaviour may be developed. For example, if the gaining of attention is the consequence of stuttering for someone, then other behaviour may be developed to produce this consequence if stuttering were eliminated. He says there are three steps to be taken when designing a treatment programme: (i) isolate the reinforcer; (ii) let the person have it; (iii) make it the consequence of the behaviour one wants the person to develop.

As part of a long-term investigation using a different approach, Goldiamond (1965) "shaped" a new form of speech in stutterers with delayed auditory feedback (DAF). Goldiamond's stutterers first developed a new speech pattern produced by the DAF. When this pattern was well established, it was "shaped" by having the stutterers speed up their speech to normal and supernormal rates. They then "observed" their speech patterns and used them outside the clinical setting while analysing the relations between their behaviour and the conditions in their environment. Finally, they were instructed to change the environment "in a manner likely to optimize the desired changes in their behaviour". This is a fairly complex example of "shaping". More usually one aspect of the final desired response is reinforced and then gradually more and more characteristics of the final response are required before reinforcement is given. A grunt from a child who will not speak at all may be reinforced at the start of the shaping procedure, but later a sound approximating a word will be required, then a recognizable word, then several words, then sentences and so on. It does seem that in some cases this procedure can produce fluency, or at least a reduction in stuttering, in some people.

Webster (1970) applied a modification of Goldiamond's approach to eight stutterers over a period of from ten to forty hours. Ten months after treatment ceased, all eight had maintained fluent speech. Once again details of the speech of these people is almost non-existent. All the information provided is the percentage of words stuttered during reading.

Another modification of Goldiamond's use of DAF to reduce stuttering has been described by Curlee and Perkins (1969). Instead of using reading as the basis of speech change, they used conversational speech and called their method Conversational Rate Control Therapy. When the speech shows no evidence of stuttering and has been reduced to the desired rate, the DAF interval is reduced until there is no delay at all. Further procedures are followed until no stuttering occurs. The stutterer is then placed in situations of increasing social complexity outside the laboratory. Curlee reports that so far fourteen adolescent or adult stutterers achieved normal conversational speech in the laboratory in less than thirty hours of treatment. There are no data available for those who have been given the "social complexity successive approximation procedures" but considerable reduction in stuttering is reported.

Shames *et al.* (1969) present a programme for modifying stuttering in a conversational setting by using social reinforcement. In this setting the clinician is seen as the instrument controlling the rewards and punishments consequent upon the stutterer's speech. These authors consider there to be two general types of stutterer; one who suffers an impairment of communication, the other who "is distinguished primarily by thematic content of his speech".

The first programme is based on the teaching of a speech modification procedure and the reinforcement of this modified speech when it occurs in the desired form. The more nearly the stutterer approaches fluency, the more nearly "normal" the speech must be to obtain the clinician's approval.

The second programme is based on the notion that "it is possible that stuttering may be maintained to a great degree because of the concepts that stutterers possess". The authors identify two broad categories of theme in the conversation of stutterers which they think are characteristic: (i) positive responses (beneficial to therapeutic success) and (ii) negative responses (incompatible with fluency). The aim of the programme is to increase the former and decrease the latter. Examples of positive responses are: "statements which reflect client's awareness or growing awareness of events or situations which accompany his stuttering or fluency" and "statements which describe a client's overt motor struggle behaviour when speaking". Examples of negative responses are "statements referring to speech or stuttering which are imprecise, vague or nondescriptive; must contain the key words *it, this*, or *this thing*". Reinforcement is given or withheld appropriately for the two types of response.

Brief data from four stutterers are given and show that positive theme responses do increase with social approval (such as "I understand", "good") and negative themes decrease with disapproval (such as "I don't agree", "I don't understand"). However, the relationship between this change and the speech change is not so clear.

The authors point out that these programmes are still very much in the experimental stage but feel that the methods of quantification may be applicable to other clinical efforts "regardless of theoretical orientation", and that they permit the clinician to relate behaviour of the client directly to his or her own behaviour.

In an attempt to assess the comparative efficacy of two treatment approaches, Martin and Haroldson (1969) had two groups of ten stutterers, each having eight sessions of either "information–attitude" therapy or "time-out from speaking" conditioning. The former procedure is basically aimed at increasing the stutterer's awareness of and knowledge about his defect, while the latter consists of having the stutterer remain silent for ten seconds after each stutter. The "information–attitude" group did not change significantly in number of disfluencies, whereas the conditioning group showed a significant reduction from first to eighth session but this reduction disappeared after two weeks. The authors emphasize the short treatment time used and suggest the conditioning procedure might form part of a more comprehensive treatment schedule, including procedures "to assist in carry-over, to bring out more desirable attitude, to increase total speaking time, to evaluate difficult or feared speaking situations more realistically, etc."

Ingham and Andrews (1972c) attempt to come to grips with a very fundamental problem in the use of techniques based on the manipulation of speech; this concerns the *quality* of the speech that has been exchanged for the stuttered speech. They point out that "a single repetition, without tension can be normal when speech is casual but in the treatment situation this type of error is regarded as a stutter. The effortless repetition of a syllable at normal speech tempo differs in quality from the tension-filled block of effortful prolongation which completely alters the flow of speech". Clearly, one or two severe blocks in five minutes' speech accompanied by obvious effort to get the speech going again on the part of the speaker shows him to be a stutterer, but in assessment these would usually only get the same score as two repetitions of syllables unaccompanied by effort and which would be regarded as part of normal speech.

Ingham and Andrews therefore looked at the form of speech at the end of treatment in those who had had syllable-timed speech and those who had received two types of auditory feedback. The former were shown to have more severe residual stutters and to speak more slowly than the latter. The authors conclude that the stutterer who is treated by syllable-timed speech is left with a slow rate of speaking which, when he tries to increase it, is likely to produce an increase in stuttering. Those receiving treatments using some form of auditory feedback had no such apparent limitations of their speed of speech.

This study goes some way toward teasing out the factors, other than stuttering itself, that make speech appear normal or abnormal to the ear of the listener. Many treatments have used methods of speech manipulation which give rise to impressive decreases in the number of disfluencies but one is left wondering how far the stutterer has swapped one form of abnormal speech for another.

A Conditioning Double. An amalgamation of the reciprocal inhibition and the operant approach has been practiced by several therapists but they are linked theoretically by Brutten and Shoemaker (1967). The therapy stemming from the theory they call Inhibition Therapy. The first phase of treatment involves taking a variety of physiological and speech measures. Systematic desensitization as previously described is then used to inhibit the anxiety reactions to a number of situations. The stutterer is taught to relax and then is encouraged to "live through" situations that normally produce anxiety. With continuing desensitization, some of the session is then spent in the "massed evocation of specific instrumental behaviours. Generally, behaviours which tend to produce punitive responses from the environment". That is, the stutterer deliberately practices certain bits of behaviour over and over again. These two procedures are co-ordinated outside the clinical room at a later stage.

This form of therapy stems from the theoretical position that (1) stuttering is the disintegration of speech fluency that results from classically conditioned negative emotion, and (2) responses of avoidance and escape are the instrumentally conditioned attempts at adjusting to anticipated, or coping with existent, punishing consequences that may be associated with stuttering.

Once again it is unfortunately impossible to assess the effects of this approach since no detailed data are given by Brutten and Shoemaker on the results of the use of this procedure with their thirty stutterers. But they do report that there is marked improvement in most of them.

C. SPEECH THERAPY OR PSYCHOTHERAPY?

While Shames and his colleagues mention the importance of the concepts the stutterer possesses, Cooper and Cooper (1969) studied the variation in feelings about the clinician during treatment, and noted that these fluctuated significantly during the four stages of their Interpersonal Communication Therapy (Cooper, 1965). In a further study (Manning and Cooper, 1969) results suggest that these patterns of affect fluctuation might be related to progress in therapy.

There is increasing emphasis on the interdependence of stutter and stutterer and that a concerted attack on both is what is required for any successful therapy. It is not thought sufficient to remove the speech defect; one has also to help the stutterer to adjust or change his attitudes to himself and others.

Van Riper was one of the early exponents of this dual approach; he basically sought to reduce the anxieties the stutterer had about speech and to simplify the stuttering pattern of speech. The stutterer is encouraged to speak whenever possible without fear, using any form of speech that he has available until he has said what he wants to say. He learns to tolerate his speech and is encouraged progressively to enter more and more difficult situations until he can enter these without anxiety even though stuttering still occurs. He is encouraged to view the situation objectively. In addition to anxiety reduction, and the re-assessment of attitudes, methods for the voluntary control of speech are taught. Van Riper describes methods which he terms "cancellation" and "pull outs". As a result of these two assaults on the speech defect, the stutterer is in the position of stuttering so little that it has ceased to be a problem. Van

Riper (1958) gives an account of how his treatment approach developed over many years. He reports his attempts to follow-up his patients and how many of them were lost by the wayside. Although the speech assessments were subjective, his description of therapeutic successes and failures is unrivalled in its detail.

Sheehan (1954) has also put the case for an integration of speech therapy and psychotherapy, linking therapy with his approach-avoidance theory of stuttering. He states that:

> Words fears and situation fears and the attitudes surrounding them are the concern of speech therapy . . .
> If the stutterer blocks more in certain necessary life roles, e.g. in the presence of father figures, he needs to find new and more satisfactory relationships with such figures. So long as the stutterer has defensive needs, and is affected in these ways, he can profit from psychotherapy. (Sheehan, 1954.)

Sheehan underlines one of the difficulties experienced in reading about and evaluating different therapies. What many people call speech therapy others would not hesitate to call psychotherapy. "The stutterer who is able to receive what speech therapy offers undergoes a profound psychotherapeutic experience."

Sheehan's (1970) own form of treatment concentrates on role-taking. He arrives at this position by combining "a role-theory with a double approach-avoidance conflict model". He argues that the presence or absence of stuttering is dependent upon how the person views his own status in a speech situation (the self variable) and how he perceives the listener (the role variable). For instance, "in a situation where the speaker role is subordinated and the self is brought forward more positively, stuttering is likely to decrease". Based on the notion that people are changed by what they do rather than what they think about or talk about, the therapy is active in that the stutterer is given specific assignments to carry out relating to his attitudes and his stuttering behaviour. Substantial reduction in stuttering has been reported using this Role Therapy programme (Gregory, 1969).

Sheehan's theoretical approach and the therapy derived from it bears some resemblance to that put forward in this present work, but at least one very basic difference is apparent. Thinking and action are here considered to be inextricably entwined. No one can act in a mental vacuum since our actions are determined by how we view a situation, and how we view the next situation will be determined by how we interpreted the previous one. Thus, change comes about both by our thinking and accepting the possibility of conducting a new behavioural experiment *and* by our putting this experiment into action. Further change will depend on the perceived outcome of the previous experiment and so on.

D. CONCLUSIONS

The last ten years has seen a considerable increase in attempts to apply theoretical principles to the treatment of stuttering. These, for the most part, have been learning theory models used in conjunction with some device to break up the existing speech pattern. But in nearly every research report there are indications that the stutterers have been helped with their "adjustment problems", however behavioural the treatment may seem. Others such as Sheehan, have used the learning theory model in conjunction with a cognitive model focusing, in Sheehan's case, on the notion of role relationships. It can be argued that a learning theory treatment of stuttering is only a partial theory if it cannot also embrace changes in thinking that take place. Beech puts the case thus:

> The tendency to disregard internal events has been the behaviour therapist's heritage; indeed it was dissatisfaction with the inadequacies of other psychological approaches, which tended to emphasize the importance of hidden processes, thus defying experimental analysis, that serves as the impetus to behaviouristic psychology. Of course, it is one thing to abandon 'mentation' as a barren field for experimental attack, and quite another to assume that cognitive processes are irrelevant to the explanation of human behaviour. In fact, the behaviour psychologist has been forced more and more, by the inadequacies of theories based solely upon overt responses, to modify and extend his conceptual analysis so that it embraces the previously taboo territories. (Beech, 1969, p. 227.)

The realization of the importance of thought process as well as the behavioural response led Kelly (1955) to describe man as a total person; his thinking, behaving and feeling are all part and parcel of how he views, interprets or construes the world around him. It is from this theoretical position that the present view of stuttering stems and which dictated the line of treatment followed.

Section II

Theory

CHAPTER 3

Personal Construct Theory

A good psychological theory has an appropriate focus and range of convenience. It suffers in usefulness when it has been transplanted from one realm to another—as, for example, from physiology to psychology. It should be fertile in producing new ideas, in generating hypotheses, in provoking experimentation, in encouraging inventions. The hypotheses which are deduced from it should be brittle enough to be testable, though the theory itself may be cast in more resilient terms. The more frequently its hypotheses turn out to be valid, the more valuable the theory.

A good psychological theory should be expressed in terms of abstractions which can be traced through most of the phenomena with which psychology must deal. In this connection, operationalism, when applied to theory construction, may interfere with the psychologist's recognition of the abstractive implications of his experimental results—he may become a laboratory technician rather than a scientist.

A psychological theory should be considered ultimately expendable. The psychologist should therefore maintain personal independence of his theory. Even experimental results never conclusively prove a theory to be ultimately true. Hypotheses are always related to some theoretical structures, but psychologists may produce them by induction or by dragnet procedures, as well as by deduction.

G. A. Kelly (1955)

I. Its Philosophy

Kelly (1955) was concerned with man the answer-seeker; with man who strives to make sense of the world around him by setting up hypotheses and putting them to experimental test. Sometimes the answer is one he expects, sometimes he gets an unpleasant surprise. But man is not at the mercy of the existential moment, since he carries around with him a system of ideas (constructs) which he has built up over the years. Nor is man a prisoner of his past, as there are always other pathways along which he can move so as to see himself in a new light. Bannister and Fransella say that:

The cardinal quality of personal construct theory is its recognition that psychology is man's understanding of his own understanding. By making its model man 'man the scientist/psychologist' it presents us with a framework which is cousin to history and poetry, while embodying the kind of systematic attack, public definition and experimental articulation which are the universal aspects of science. It is a psychological theory which admits that values are implicit in all psychological theories and takes as its own central concern the liberation of the person. (Bannister and Fransella, 1971, p. 12.)

Kelly called his philosophical position *Constructive Alternativism*, that is:

> We assume that all our present interpretations of the universe are subject to revision or replacement . . . We take the stand that there are always some alternative constructions available to choose among in dealing with the world, no one needs to paint himself into a corner; no one needs to be completely hemmed in by circumstances; no one needs to be the victim of his biography. (Kelly, 1955, p. 15.)

II. The Construct System

The central idea in personal construct theory is stated in its fundamental postulate: *a person's processes are psychologically channelized by the ways in which he anticipates events*. This postulate is elaborated by eleven corollaries and each word of each corollary is defined, making it one of the most explicit theoretical systems in psychology to-day.

The basis of these anticipations is the *construct*. These have evolved through our seeing certain similarities and contrasts in happenings in our environment. Kelly gives the example of how noting the rise of the sun in the morning and its setting in the evening enables us to construe *day*. Having construed the replication of solar events in this way, we can predict that to-morrow will be similar to to-day *in that* the sun will rise in the morning and set in the evening, and will *differ from* to-day in weather, events, feelings of personal well-being and what we have for supper.

All constructs are dichotomous; we cannot know what *day* is if we do not have something such as *night* with which to contrast it, nor black without white. Constructs are seen as being linked so as to form a hierarchical system; some constructs are more subordinate than others, some more superordinate; some form themselves into sub-systems and some vary according to the context in which they are applied. Being linked into a system, the use of one construct implies the relevance of several others. For instance, to construe an event as *a horse race* implies the probability of losing money, of horses taking their jockeys around in a circle before the race starts, and a group of men using a unique language system. Before going to a particular horse race we can predict that certain events will happen, in common with other horse races, and that certain events will be different.

Hinkle (1965) places great emphasis on the context in which constructs are used to anticipate events. "What a person considers to be 'honest' in the context of criminals may be vastly different from 'honest' in the context of intimate friends." This comment highlights the fact that one should never equate the construct with its verbal label. The *commonality corollary* suggests that people in a given culture will tend to use many constructs in a similar way, while the *individuality corollary* says that people differ from each other in their construction of events. When people use the construct *honest*, many of its implications will be held in common by two people from a similar culture, yet we cannot assume that these implications are identical for these two people. The mistaken belief that the identical verbal label indicates the use of an identical construct can often be seen in discussions. All is going smoothly until one discussant falters. The careful listener can sometimes discern a conflict between the implications of the constructs being used (particularly at a superordinate or abstract level) the discussants have ceased to "speak the same language". Two people may construe stutterers as *shy*, but for person "A" this means being *uninteresting* and *stupid* whereas for person "B" this means being *interesting* because the stutterer is *not showing his true self* which means there is *a great deal still to be found out about him*—whether he is *stupid* or *clever* is immaterial.

Construct systems relating to people reflect the values each culture places on certain personality characteristics. To be a *nice* man in one culture is to be *quiet*, someone who *always puts people at their ease* and who has a *generous heart*; whereas to be construed as having a *strong personality*, as being a *leader* and someone who *thirsts for power and knowledge* is to be *scorned* and *disliked*. Another culture may have the reverse view. Thus, the "ideal" man and his opposite are central features in determining how an individual thinks and behaves towards others in a given culture.

III. Some Theoretical Constructs

A. ROLE

If one had lived at the time of P. G. Woodhouse's Bertie Wooster and had hesitations in his speech, this would have been construed as evidence of his occupying a certain place in the social hierarchy in which a speech impediment was fashionable—to-day the same person might well be categorized as a stutterer. In construct theory terms, Bertie Wooster was playing a role in relation to his listeners. Kelly has a slightly unusual notion of role. It stems from his *sociality corollary*, which states that *to the extent that one person construes the construction processes of another, he may play a role in the social process involving the other person*. Bertie Wooster understood the construction processes of his listener and knew that he would not be construed as a stutterer but as one coming from a certain stratum of society. Role, for Kelly, is thus not a course of action in relation to others nor is it a set of expectations held by others which places limitations of an individual's possible courses of action. Instead, it is:

A psychological process based upon the role player's construction of aspects of the construction systems of those whom he attempts to join in a social enterprise. In less precise but more familiar language, a role is an ongoing pattern of behaviour that follows from a person's understanding of how the others who are associated with him in his task think. In idiomatic language, a role is a position that one can play on a certain team without even waiting for the signals. (Kelly, 1955, p. 97.)

B. RANGE OF CONVENIENCE

Other important corollaries deal with such notions as *range of convenience*. Some constructs can be used to help us make sense of a very large number of events, such as the dimension *beautiful-ugly*, while others have a very limited range of applicability, such as *draught-bottled*, which can be used to construe beers or ciders but little else. Sometimes a person can himself apply a construct to such a narrow range of events that it is of little real use to him. Or sometimes the opposite occurs, he uses a construct dimension to make sense of almost everything that happens to him. Some theories are applicable to a very narrow range of events while others can be applied very extensively—such as construct theory. Theories not only have a range of convenience, but also a focus of convenience. The focus for a theory is the area where it works best, and for construct theory this is "the area of human adjustment to stress".

C. EMOTIONS

It has often been said that Kelly's theory is too cognitive—too many ideas chasing too little action—and that it allows too little scope for the concept of emotion. It is true that Kelly redefined such terms as anxiety, hostility, threat, guilt and aggression, but he did not say that what *he* called anxiety was thereby different from what everyone else called anxiety. If one feels his heart beating rapidly, is sweating together with a churning over of the stomach prior to taking an examination, this will be, in construct theory terms, because one is faced with the recognition that *the events with which one is confronted lie outside the range of convenience of one's construct system.*

In the first major extension of Kelly's theoretical system, Hinkle (1965) redefined anxiety in terms of his theory of construct implications to read *anxiety is the awareness of the relative absence of implications with respect to the constructs with which one is confronted*. It is the construing of failure that is the problem. The construing of oneself at the *failure* end of the *success–failure* dimension has relatively few implications compared with the meaningfulness of being a success. It is always very important to remember that, in theoretical terms, construing does not have to take place at the conscious level. Constructs are discriminations which can be applied to aspects of the environment at a cognitive, psychological, emotional or behavioural level. Discriminations *need not necessarily* be verbalized.

Closely related to the concept of anxiety is the notion of *threat*. Threat is *the awareness of imminent comprehensive change in one's core structures*; or in Hinkle's terms *the awareness of an imminent comprehensive reduction of the total number of predictive implications of the personal construct system*. The student who goes home for the holidays could be threatened if his parents refused to acknowledge by their behaviour that he is now a grown-up individual and insist on treating him like a child. A stutterer may be threatened when approaching fluency if he meets people who have only known him as a stutterer and expect him to behave as one.

Guilt is defined as *the perception of one's apparent dislodgement from his core role structure*. The woman who sees herself as primarily the *mother*, may experience guilt when her children grow up and leave home. She has never developed an alternative core role and so she finds herself being a *mother* without any "mothering" to do.

Another of Kelly's redefinitions concerns the notion of *hostility*. This he defines as *the continued effort to extort validational evidence in favour of a type of social prediction which has already proved itself a failure*. The student goes home and rejects his new-found ways of independence and adopts those child-like ways of old; his parents react to him *as if* he were a child. He is then able to turn round and berate them for "always treating me like a child and that is why I do not like to come home often". Bannister and Fransella (1971) have argued that prejudiced thinking can lead to Kellian hostility. Prejudiced thinking is seen as characterized by the use of constellatory and pre-emptive constructs; the former construing is of the "if a man is french *he must also be* sexy, untrustworthy and shrewd"-type. Pre-emptive construing is of the "if this is a french-man he is *nothing but* a frenchman—he cannot simultaneously be construed as a sportsman, an economist or a father-in-law"-type. These authors go on to say that:

> The second characteristic of prejudiced thinking, in construct theory terms, arises from the linked notions of core constructs and hostility. It seems likely that for each of us our prejudiced ideas are core ideas, they involve dimensions along which we choose to see ourselves and others most significantly—they refer to maintenance processes. Thus, any invalidation of our expectations in terms of those constructs would imply the need for a major revision of our outlook, a revision for which we may be ill-prepared. If these core ideas are experienced as being less meaningful, then we are threatened, we are made aware of "imminent comprehensive change in our structures" ... Our reactions to such potential chaos is almost inevitably hostility, we refuse to be wrong, we set out to extort validational evidence for our prejudices, we cook the books, we deny the validity of the source of contradictory evidence. (Bannister and Fransella, 1971, p. 112.)

5

As well as redefining some popular but multi-defined terms, Kelly has had the audacity to "eliminate" whole areas of psychology, such as learning. This does not mean that he denied that people "learn", but rather that one does not need a separate heading for this particular form of construing. Learning as a concept is rendered redundant by the *experience corollary* which states that *a person's construction system varies as he successively construes the replication of events.*

Another example of Kelly's dissatisfaction with some existing psychological concepts is his rejection of the concept of motivation. Like so many other concepts in psychology, this was "borrowed" from the physical sciences. Matter is basically inert and, therefore, something has to make it move. For the psychologist, man is usually seen as either driven from within or responding in a rather rigid way to stimuli that impinge on his senses from without. But Kelly (1962) says "suppose we began by assuming that the fundamental thing about life is that it goes on. It is not that motives *make* man come alert and do things; his alertness is an aspect of his very being". Man is thus an on-going process. To find out why he does A rather than B and hopefully to try and predict what he may do in the future, one studies the ways in which he views and interprets events in the world around him.

D. PERSONALITY

From the construct theory standpoint, a man's personality is his total view of himself, his life and his world. How he reacts to his world is totally dependent upon his view of that world. This approach differs in a very fundamental way from those theories of personality which describe man in terms of traits, such as extraversion versus introversion or dominance versus submission. It differs also from theories in which a person's thinking and behaviour are forced into slots conceived of by others, such as when a boy's aggressive feelings for his father are interpreted as being the result of an unresolved oedipus complex. For construct theory, the man himself does his own interpreting of what he sees whether it be something in his own actions or in the actions of others. His interpretation may not always be a very good fit on the events, but he is seen as constantly trying to live consistently in terms of his view of the world. In these terms, a man's personality and his construct system are synonymous.

IV. PSYCHOLOGICAL CHANGE

By forming his constructs into a system, man interprets events in his world, makes predictions which subsequent events will prove right or wrong. It is the understanding of this construct system that is the aim of psychotherapy or "the reconstruction process". Kelly says he would have preferred not to have to use the term "psychotherapy" because of its implications of underlying illness or disease.

> Since we see processes psychologically channelized by one's construction system, we can view them as being changed either by re-routing through the same system of dichotomous constructs, or by reconstruction of the system of channels . . . we see (the latter) as the ultimate objective of the clinical-psychological enterprise and we have used it as the basis for the theme of this book—*The Psychological Reconstruction of Life*. We even considered using the term *reconstruction* instead of therapy. If it had not been such a mouth-filling word we might have gone ahead with the idea. Perhaps later we may! (Kelly, 1955, p. 187.)

Psychotherapy traditionally involves the idea of two people getting together in an attempt to solve the problem of one of them. The implication being that one of them is in a specially good position, on account of training or experience, to help the other. This does not rule out the priest or the best friend; the former having particular experience of the difficulties people can get themselves into and the best friend having particular experience and knowledge of the one in trouble. Psychotherapy differs in that there is an attempt to apply specific principles, derived theoretically or empirically, to bring about psychological change in a person. The term psychotherapy also often implies a second factor, the use of concepts concerning illness. Psychotherapists are usually psychiatrists (thus medically trained) who apply notions of disease to a problem and establish the doctor–patient relationship. However, there is no good reason why this should be so and many of those in other professions (e.g. psychologists and speech pathologists) practice what looks, to all intents and purposes, like psychotherapy, but do not necessarily subscribe to the 'illness model'. The problem is, what does one call the attempt by one person to "change" aspects of another if one does not see disorders in terms of disease? Behaviour therapists may use the terms deconditioning or behaviour modification; others use words like retraining or re-education; Kelly suggests the term reconstruction.

Whether one word will be found to stand in contrast to the term psychotherapy, or whether each theoretical approach will coin a word of its own, remains to be seen. The construct theory position is that the use of the medical concept in relation to psychological difficulties is not only unnecessary, but is far too limiting a frame of reference. Kelly puts it thus:

> . . . the term "therapy" and its companion term "patient" carry many implications which we are reluctant to buy. Most of all, they carry the implication that the person served is reduced to an ultimate state of passivity

and that his recovery depends upon his submitting *patiently* and unquestioningly to the manipulations of a clinician. We think this is a badly misleading view of how a psychologically disturbed person recovers. (Kelly, 1955, p. 186.)

He goes on to say that he uses Rogers' term "Client" instead of "Patient" but that "we have submitted to the term 'therapy', even though what we mean by 'therapy' is quite different from what is commonly called 'therapy' ". The term will be used in the report to follow on the application of construct theory to bring about change from stutterer to fluent speaker. This is to facilitate communication and does not imply that stutterers are viewed as patients and therefore in some way are psychologically ill. The path from stuttering to fluency is seen as being by a process of *reconstruction*.

CHAPTER 4

A Personal Construct Theory of Stuttering

Specialization is in the saddle. Bad enough is the parochialism resulting from traditional national cleavages (an anachronism in a shrunken world). Much worse is the fact that theorizing, especially in the grand manner, is frowned out of court in psychology—though not in other sciences. Conant (1951) tells us that the course of science is toward larger and larger abstractions. Psychology seems headed in the opposite direction. Miniscule theories we have, but scarcely any that are comprehensively human in their reference.

The Fruits of Eclecticism—Bitter or Sweet?
Gordon W. Allport (1964)

I. GENERAL STATEMENT

Deliberately contravening Kelly's basic philosophical statement *we assume that all of our present interpretations of the universe are subject to revision or replacement*, the pre-emptive view is taken here that *man is nothing but a bundle of constructs*. Rejected is the idea that man is driven by unconscious forces; is a black box responding automatically to the environment because of pairings of conditioned stimuli or schedules of reinforcement; is a computer with spongy parts; or seeks experience for its own sake.

These are all constructive alternatives but for present purposes the model is *man the construer*. Man sometimes stutters and stutterers construe. They, like all men, have developed sub-systems of constructs through which to view the universe of events that confront them and hope to predict and hence control the course of these events. When our predictions are not borne out or are invalidated, there are several possible courses of action open to us. We might modify our predictions and put them to the test again to see if they are more accurate a second time; we might stick to our guns and say we misread the evidence; or we might "fix" the evidence and so show *hostility* (in the Kellian sense).

Our construct systems make us both free men and prisoners. We are free in that we can change our construing of events in the light of the results of our predictions. But we are trapped by this same construing system. We have a choice, but we can only choose between the dichotomous constructs that make up our system; we cannot view the world along totally new construct dimensions at will. The choice corollary suggests that we choose the alternative pole in a dichotomous construct which will give us the greatest possibility for extension and definition of our system. Hinkle (1965) has worded the corollary in a slightly different form: "a person always chooses in that direction which he anticipates will increase the total meaning and significance of his life. Stated in the defensive form, a person chooses so as to avoid the anxiety of chaos and the despair of absolute certainty".

It is argued that *a person stutters because it is in this way that he can anticipate the greatest number of events: it is by behaving in this way that life is most meaningful to him*. He has constructs which enable him to anticipate or make predictions about himself and others. He chooses those poles of his constructs which provide him with the best predictive possibilities. He does not change his stance because none of us willingly walks the plank and so drops off into an unknown, unpredictable world. In the world of fluency there lie many unknown hazards and a vastly decreased ability to predict these pitfalls.

Stuttering in adults occurs nearly always in verbal communication with other adults. Bloodstein (1949) concluded, after surveying the literature, that stuttering is less likely to occur when the person talks to animals, children, or to himself, when he recites something he has learned or is acting a part. In fact, stuttering seems to be likely in almost any situation in which there is little necessity to communicate information or in which the stutterer is not being "himself". Talking to adults is when the stutterer's predictive problem is at its more difficult and he therefore adopts the most familiar, the most meaningful, mode for understanding and managing other people. The very complexity of the situation forces him to stutter.

The stutterer knows all about playing the "stutterer" role (in the Kellian sense); he knows the variety of ways in which a person will react to his speaking, and knows what his reactions will be to the listener's reactions. But he is inexperienced at interpreting the subtler forms of communication such as eye contacts, hand gestures and general body movements, which are normal reactions to the fluent person. His focus of attention is mainly on himself, on the degree of difficulty he is having in getting out the words he wants, and he is busy interpreting the reactions of the listener, which on most occasions are reactions *to him as a stutterer*. When he speaks he construes himself as a stutterer.

II. Construct Sub-systems

The stutterer is seen as having a sub-system of constructs to do with himself as a communicator. This has been built up within the speaking context and involves certain role relationships (*to the extent that one person construes the construction processes of another, he may play a role in a social process involving the other person*). The stutterer can read the signs and "knows" what another thinks of him and "knows" what sort of reactions he may get. He "knows" that he is unlikely to be interrupted, to be shouted at, even, in many cases, to be disagreed with; he easily holds the listener's attention, albeit unwillingly.

As individuals we adopt many roles depending upon the context in which we find ourselves. At a cocktail party we may be the "bright young thing" or the "man of the world" and modify our behaviour according to the reactions we get. Some people try to be "all things to all men", while others are severely limited in the roles they have available. In effect, the sociality corollary of construct theory:

> ... sees each of us as attempting, in relation to other people, to be psycho-logists—whether we be good, bad or indifferent psychologists. In terms of our ideas about the other person's construct system we may seek to inspire the other person, confuse him, amuse him, change him, win his affection, help him to pass the time of day or defeat him. But in all these and many other ways we are playing a role in a social process with him. (Bannister and Fransella, 1971, p. 31).

The stutterer gets little opportunity to construe the construction processes of others in relation to himself except when in the role of a stutterer —he is a psychologist with but a single thought. Many stutterers have an increase in fluency as their knowledge of the other person increases. There tends to be less likelihood of stuttering with friends, husbands, wives, boy friends or girl friends. With repeated social interactions these stutterers are able to construe some aspects of the other's construct system and so find no desperate need to act as stutterers. That disfluencies are dependent upon the constructions one places on situations has been demonstrated by Broen and Siegel (1972). From a study of normal speakers they conclude that "the important generalization would appear to be that, regardless of the particular situation, if the subject regards it as one in which it is important to speak carefully, he will be relatively fluent".

Some stutterers appear to adopt roles on the basis of stereotyped construing, such as in terms of sex or social class. Stereotypes, in construct theory terms, can be considered the equivalent of construing in a constellatory and pre-emptive fashion. Stereotyped "social class" construing, for example, might be such that "this person is a *social inferior*, he must therefore be *unintelligent, lacking in drive*, and *not deserving of respect*". A stutterer may have less difficulty in speaking with this person, construed as *socially inferior*, but much more difficulty with another designated as *socially superior* because he can be less easily construed stereotypically. This same stutterer may equally well be fluent with a girl because he has learned how to interpret some of the "sex" cues. But where he is unable to construe the construction processes of others, even if only in a stereotyped way, he has to fall back on the one role he knows all too well—that of the stutterer.

The stutterer is thus seen as having a very limited repertoire of ways of reacting to people he cannot adequately construe. The only way he can start to build up a repertoire of roles is by dropping his stuttering and experimenting with being a fluent speaker. Once he need not be concerned with *disfluent* speech he can experiment in social relationships to his heart's content, or at least until he gets some answers he does not particularly like. (Fransella, 1969, 1970a, 1971b.)

III. Some Construct Theory Corollaries

The fragmentation corollary states that *a person may successively employ a variety of construct sub-systems which are inferentially incompatible with each other*. Hinkle suggests that 'inferential incompatibilities will be resolved only when such a resolution is anticipated to maximize the total implicativeness of the personal construct system.' In the present construct theory approach to stuttering this means that a person can maintain a construct sub-system relating to *himself as a stuttering speaker* which contradicts many ideas he has about *himself as a person*. Such inferential incompatibility is suggested by the finding that in all the ninety-three implications grids completed by the stutterers in the present research, only five showed a significant positive relationship between the constructs *like me in character* and *stutterers*; the most severe stutterer had a significant *negative* correlation—he was definitely *not* like other stutterers. Additional evidence of incompatibility in the construing of the self can be seen in Fig. 1 (p. 24), where the idea of the self and that of being a stutterer occupy very different positions along the two dimensions of meaning for each of the three groups (stutterers, male and female nonstutterers). Figure 3 (p. 26) shows the different "meanings" given to these two constructs by one stutterer.

It is argued that a stutterer will only give up this sub-system, which is in some respects incompatible with the rest of his self construing system, if, by doing so, he is able to *see* that he is likely to make the whole system generally a more meaningful proposition. In his present state, to suddenly become a fluent person would be to deny himself the one role in which he has become expert and which at least enables him to extract some meaning from inter-personal relationships.

The range corollary. This notion of the "stutterer" sub-system is *convenient for the anticipation of a finite range of events only*. That is, it applies only to situations involving the imparting of information to certain types of people, for example, adult humans as opposed to children and animals.

The individuality corollary. Stutterers differ from each other in their construction of events. Some men can speak fluently to girls, perhaps because they can construe them stereotypically as *kind, friendly, sympathetic* creatures, while others cannot, perhaps instead construing them as *birds of prey, liable to pounce and emasculate any man who cannot demonstrate his masculinity.* It must be remembered that how a person (stutterer or not) construes a situation determines how he behaves in that situation. Kelly says that "it is possible for two people to be involved in the same real events but, because they construe them differently, to experience them differently. Since they construe them differently, they will anticipate them differently and will behave differently as a consequence of their anticipations." (p. 90).

The commonality corollary. This states that *to the extent that one person employs a construction of experience which is similar to that employed by another, his psychological processes are similar to those of the other person.* Just as stutterers differ from each other in many ways, so they construe some events in similar fashion. They need not have had similar experience, but just to have construed certain events in a similar way. There are many ways, for instance, of construing "authority", but the expectations of many stutterers vis à vis authority are similar and these expectations often lead to increased stuttering.

A simple investigation of the commonality of some constructs for the group of stutterers and some used in an individual way is described in Chapter 8. For instance, situations construed as anxiety-provoking or as those in which it is difficult to see or interpret others' reactions, were construed by the group as likely to produce increased stuttering, while situations construed as producing a feeling of confidence were seen as less likely to evoke stuttering. On the other hand, whereas for the majority, talking to men was construed as more difficult than talking to women, for one person this process was reversed. The results were much as would be expected, but serve to show the application of the individuality and commonality corollaries in quantitative terms.

IV. Stuttering and Emotions

A. STUTTERING AND ANXIETY

One of the most frequent observations about stutterers is that their behaviour seems to cause them considerable emotional discomfort, usually described as "anxiety". As has already been mentioned, Kelly defined the term anxiety so as to incorporate it within the framework of his theory of personal constructs. Hinkle later redefined it as *the awareness of the relative absence of implications with respect to the constructs with which one is confronted.* At first sight this looks like a direct contradiction of the theory that people stutter because this is the most meaningful way of behaving *for them*. But it has been argued that the stutterer has developed a construct sub-system within the *context* of verbal communication. There is some evidence that this *me as a speaker* sub-system is dissimilar to the construing of the self in other contexts. If the *me as a speaker* sub-system is viewed as one part of the total construct system, then every time he plays the stutterer role he is aware of the relative absence of implications of this role in relation to his total system.

Further, the more he construes a situation as *important* (the more it involves superordinate construing), the more aware he becomes of the impoverishment of his stuttering posture. But equally, the more vital it becomes for him to hang on to whatever meaningful construing he has and so the likelihood of his stuttering is increased. He is virtually forced to stutter to gain control of the situation in which he is anxious (confronted by elements which he is not well able to construe). The more anxious he is, the more likely he is to stutter because in this way he turns the situation into one that he well understands and in which he can make predictions. Conversely, when he can well construe the other person's reactions he is not anxious (in the Kellian sense) and therefore does not stutter. He is obliged to introduce stuttering (and so gain control by altering the tone of the communication to one which he can construe) because of the impoverishment and inadequacy of his initial construing. Only when he is able to elaborate this will he cease having to resort to stuttering.

Fluency itself is also anxiety-provoking. Sheehan (1954) comments on the observation that stutterers sometimes become very anxious if asked what difference it would make to their lives if their stuttering suddenly disappeared. To be suddenly fluent instead of stuttering would produce an immediate awareness of the relative lack of implications within the speaking situation. The aim of treatment is thus to increase the meaningfulness of being a fluent speaker and to integrate this or make it inferentially compatible with the total construct system.

B. STUTTERING AND THREAT

How threatening for the stutterer fluency must be when threat is defined as *the awareness of imminent comprehensive change in one's core structures* (Kelly, 1955) or in Hinkle's terminology *the awareness (e.g. a superordinate construction and anticipation about the construct system) of an imminent comprehensive reduction of the total number of predictive implications of the personal construct system.* In the first place, total fluency is anxiety-provoking because of the stutterer's awareness of the reduction in meaningfulness of that form of behaviour in certain situations. But as treatment progresses and reconstruing occurs, there is often an awareness of the enormity of the change that is going to take place when he truly enters the world of the fluent speaker.

It is the job of the therapist to take the stutterer along slowly enough so that he can "creep up on" fluency, a glimpse at a time. That he is going to change as he becomes more fluent is undeniable; there will be all sorts of things he will be able to do which were previously unavailable to him, new roles to adopt, new limits to impose on his behaviour. Also, with increased fluency, such events as returning home, or meeting old friends can be threatening. Kelly puts the position thus:

> Usually threat is related to "movement" or to the development of one's psychological construct system; thus, a threat is that which confronts us with the possibility that we have not really made any progress, that we are still children, that we have not really extricated ourselves from the past, that we have not really rid ourselves of undesirable characteristics, that our efforts have come to naught. (Kelly, 1955, p. 717.)

Landfield's (1954) extension of this notion of threat has possible implications for the group treatment of stutterers, and possibly for other group treatments where there is some homogeniety among the members. Landfield has experimental support for the theory that:

> Discomfort with and avoidance of another person are intimately tied to perception of one's personal change. Meeting someone, and being reminded at some level of awareness, of oneself in the recent past, produces discomfort, avoidance and possibly a desire to change the other's behaviour. Such a person is a "reminder" of the overcome past and hence is perceived as threatening, i.e. threatening to elicit regressive behaviour in oneself. (Landfield and Fjeld, 1960.)

Several instances of threat such as this, together with its relations to stuttering severity, are recorded in the detailed account of the therapeutic process in Chapter 9.

V. Aetiology

Any theory of behaviour carries with it implications for an explanation of how such behaviour developed in the first place. At this stage of knowledge, any personal construct theory of the aetiology of stuttering must be purely speculative since there has been little theorizing and there is even less experimental evidence about how construing systems develop.

One of the very few attempts to explain how the child develops his inter-personal construing centres upon Kelly's notion of role (Salmon,

1970). The child is viewed as organizing his world, however imperfectly, by seeing it through his mother's eyes. This presumably includes his mother's view of him, thus starting the development of his construing of *self*. This approach has a great deal in common with that of Johnson (1955), who argued that a child becomes a stutterer after he has been so diagnosed by someone, usually his parents. Johnson reached this conclusion after finding it very difficult to differentiate between the recorded speech of two groups of children who had been designated stutterers or nonstutterers by their parents.

Sander (1963) reports that, in his experience, mothers will talk about their child stuttering but will not willingly call him a stutterer. He describes a "linguistic evolution" in which "we begin with 'stuttering behaviour', pass first to 'behaviour which *shows* stuttering', and then to 'behaviour which occurs because the individual *is* a stutterer' ".

For Johnson, the child diagnosed as a stutterer by his parents, or whoever are the important figures in his life, will be worried about speaking, will therefore focus attention on his speech, which in turn, will result in more rather than less stuttering. But there is no experimental evidence about the relationship between anxiety and speech disfluencies in the child, and there is conflicting evidence concerning the presence of over-anxiety and perfectionism in the parents of stuttering children. For instance, Goldman and Shames (1964a, b) found that parents of child stutterers did not differ from parents of nonstuttering children in the goals they set *themselves* in a task, but they did set higher goals for their stuttering *children*. Quarrington and his co-workers (1969), on the other hand, found the opposite to be the case. However, it does seem that child stutterers do not differ from child nonstutterers in the way they perceive the behaviour of their parents (Bourdon and Silber, 1970). These authors suggest that research attention would be better directed to looking at specific behaviour, such as calling the child's attention to disfluencies or embarrassing him in some way, rather than looking for general traits in which one group differs from the other.

From the personal construct theory point of view, the focus of interest is parent/child interaction. It is not necessary to suppose that all mothers of stuttering children share certain characteristics, or that all stuttering children have some personality characteristics in common. The concern is with how the mother construes her child, for it is this that may determine how the child construes his mother, himself and the world around him. As a prototype, consider a mother who construes her relationship with her child as a "good" one, in which love and care exist and in which she is concerned to do her best for him. One of his imperfections (in her eyes) is that he stumbles too much in his speech. She may be anxious about it because Uncle Harry stuttered or she may simply be concerned that he "get it right", whatever her reason she draws his attention to his speech. The child, playing a role in relation to her as he does, construes her constructions of him and his speech. But what does he actually construe? This is a young child, the majority of whose constructions will be at the pre-verbal level; he is more likely to be making behavioural than verbal discriminations. He begins to discriminate between, say, the sounds he makes to his mother and the sounds he makes when by himself. His mother is making him construe his disfluencies, but not his fluencies. There is no need to postulate any Kellian anxiety here since the child probably does not "see" any of the implications of his mother's constructions. There is no particular reason why they should have any more meaning for him to begin with than when she calls attention to his dirty shoes or tousled hair. But by starting him off on construing his disfluencies, she has laid the basis for the development of a construct sub-system that in time *will* have implications for him.

This construct sub-system to do with speech will come to have linkages with superordinate constructs in the rest of the system and, as has been discussed in relation to the general theory, anxiety can be expected to arise when the child has a sufficiently elaborated sub-system concerning stuttering in contrast to the embryonic system for construing people when he is fluent. *The child has never been in a position to establish a network of implications to do with himself as a fluent speaker to equal that of the network to do with himself as a stuttering speaker.*

There is no reason to suppose that fluent children ever do establish a very elaborated sub-system to do with speech in the normal course of events; like other abilities such as walking, it develops without the child construing it in any detailed way. As adults we may discriminate between "our walk" and the "walks" of other people, or "our speech" and that of others but it seems likely that these are fairly rudimentary sub-systems unless, for some reason, they are important in our lives. It must be emphasized again that there is no experimental evidence whatever to support these contentions, but ideas derived from personal construct theory can be formulated in ways in which variables can be operationally defined and experimentally tested.

One further point remains to be discussed; that of the notion of the inheritability of stuttering. It is well known that girls are superior to boys in language ability during the first few years of speech development. Not only is there a difference in verbal ability between the sexes but also within the sex groups. Thus, some boys develop speech early and have few errors while others develop speech late and make many errors while doing so. It is possible that the potential stutterer is one who has a low level of language ability and also has a parent or parent figure who notices this and tries to do something about it. It is not necessary to assume that stuttering itself is part of the child's genetic make-up, but simply to assume that genetically he may be less well endowed with the ability to use words than the majority of children and that certain environmental pressures turn his disfluent speech into stuttered speech.

VI. Prognosis

Prognosis for the child stutterer is known to be good. Salmon (1970) has suggested that the child elaborates his construing system through the widening scope for role relationships. So, when the disfluent child comes into contact with other children and teachers, much will depend on how he interprets their reactions to him. If these reactions give him no cause to elaborate his "stutterer" sub-system, or if they invalidate some of his expectancies, then the "stuttering" sub-system may be expected to disintegrate or become markedly constricted from disuse.

VII. Range of Convenience of the Theory

Any theory should attempt to explain at least some of the relevant experimental findings. In the field of stuttering, many of the phenomena investigated are those pertaining to speech generally, rather than to stuttering in particular. For example, adaptation, consistency and expectancy effects are present in normal speech but are exaggerated in the stutterer because there is more scope for them to take place.

Gray (1965) has defined adaptation as a continuing adjustment process to an ongoing constant stimulus situation. The 'continuing adjustment process' is a restatement of the experience corollary of construct theory (a person's construction system varies as he successively construes the replication of events). The stutterer is normally so busy construing his speech that he has little chance to construe the reactions of others except in relation to his stuttering; he has little chance of elaborating his role construing by noting replication of events and so forth. However, in a relatively constant experimental situation, where he is required to read the same passage or say the same things over and over again, he has more of a chance. He is experiencing a *relatively* 'ongoing constant stimulus situation'. However, the other person or people present cannot but be reacting to the individual before them. So a construct theory approach would lead one to look at some of the dimensions each individual stutterer (or normal speaker) is using to construe others. Attempts could be made to predict the degree of adaptation likely to occur when reading before, say, a man, a woman, someone sympathetic, someone authoritarian, or whatever the important constructs for that individual might be.

Johnson (1955) has stated that this adaptation process is "a kind of laboratory model of the improvement process". The adaptation situation perhaps gives the stutterer time to construe. Why, then, does the reduction in stuttering disappear after a few hours? Johnson has likened the process of spontaneous recovery to a laboratory model of relapse. Kelly argues as follows:

> Experience is made up of the successive construing of events. It is not constituted merely by the succession of events themselves. A person can be a witness to a tremendous parade of episodes and yet, if he fails to keep making something out of them, or if he waits until they have all occurred before he attempts to reconstrue them, he gains little in the way of experience from having been around when they happened. It is not what happens around him that makes a man experienced; it is the successive construing and reconstruing of what happens, as it happens, that enriches the experience of his life.
>
> Our Corollary also throws emphasis upon construing the replicative features of experience. The person who merely stands agog at each emerging event may experience a series of interesting surprises, but if he makes no attempt to discover the recurrent themes, his experience does not amount to much. It is when man begins to see the orderliness in a sequence of events that he begins to experience them. (Kelly, 1955, p. 73.)

In the adaptation situation, the stutterer is construing a particular situation and fails to reconstrue in such a way that he can take advantage of his experience in the first situation and apply it when confronted with a second similar situation. For him, each adaptation situation is a "different" situation and so he starts from square one each time.

This approach leads to agreement, theoretically at least, with Johnson in emphasizing the importance of the adaptation situation in its relation to improvement. The evidence of a tendency for stutterers showing a high percentage of adaptation to have more chance of improving in therapy is equivocal (Lanyon, 1965; Prins, 1968). But if the stutterer could be made to construe the replicative themes in these situations, a basis of change from stuttering to fluency could be found.

There is ample evidence that "... the decrease in stuttering, as measured with reference to its frequency or severity, that occurs when a stutterer reads the same passage a number of times consecutively" (Johnson, 1955) occurs in the speech of nonstutterers as well (e.g. Brutten, 1963; Williams *et al.*, 1968). Williams concludes that:

> Our findings ... indicate that adaptation is not uniquely a characteristic of the disfluent behaviour of stutterers. It is a characteristic also of the disfluent behaviour of normal speakers. Whether or not an individual exhibits this phenomenon appears to be more closely related to how disfluent he is on his

first performance of a task than to whether he has been labelled as a stutterer or a nonstutterer.

Likewise with the consistency effect. Stutterers are known to be fairly consistent in finding certain words more difficult than others (Brown, 1945; Taylor, 1966). Brown isolated four attributes of words that make them increasingly likely to lead to disfluencies: (i) words beginning with certain consonants; (ii) adjectives, nouns, adverbs or verbs; (iii) words coming first, second or third in a sentence; (iv) words of five letters or more in length. Stutterers are not alone in this. Adult and child non-stutterers are more likely to find these words more difficult (Silverman and Williams, 1967; Williams *et al.*, 1969).

Children and adults are also consistent in that they are disfluent on the same words when a speaking or reading task is repeated more than once, be they stutterer or nonstutterer (e.g. Johnson and Knott, 1937; Neelley and Timmons, 1967; Williams *et al.*, 1969). The fact that people can predict when they are going to be disfluent and are consistent in the choice of words on which they are going to be disfluent, suggests that they have construed the difficulties inherent in certain words and sentence structure. As these phenomena are not peculiar to the stutterer, they can be studied within the general context of language. If it is accepted that people can be studied as construers, then the person's construing of language is a legitimate area for study.

One further link between the disfluencies of stutterers and non-stutterers is provided by Goldman-Eisler (1958). She demonstrated that hesitations in speech are more likely to occur when people are faced with uncertainty (unpredictability); pauses tending to occur before long words, "content" words and words of high information value. Taylor (1966b) argues that:

> In stuttering, the factors of position, length, and possibly grammatical class, plus initial sound of words have been shown to affect the frequency of stuttering. These loci of greater possibility of stuttering also appear to be the loci of great uncertainty. A stutterer, just as a normal speaker, might well have trouble in speaking or reading when there are many possibilities for the next word or when constructing and formulating ideas for a sentence are involved. But where the normal speaker merely hesitates, the stutterer's speech is disrupted. (Taylor, 1966b.)

It thus looks as if a stutterer stutters whenever faced with what he cannot construe adequately—that is, what is relatively unpredictable, be it people or language. If he is seen as a person who stutters in order to gain control over (make predictable) a situation, then he has to stutter on words. It seems as if he may use the same "rules" in his choice of these as govern his choice of situations in which to stutter.

VIII. A Construct Theory Approach to Stuttering Research

The construct theory approach makes the research worker concentrate on the individual to find out how he orders his world, rather than on how he behaves in relation to it. It cannot be reiterated too often that how we construe an act, person, place or thing determines how we behave in relation to that act, person, place or thing. No situation is intrinsically dangerous, anxiety-provoking or beautiful, it is only so if we construe in that way. No particular word or situation is more "difficult" than any other unless it is so construed. Whipping may be pain for one person and ecstasy for another. From a construct theory standpoint, the study of speech can be carried out within the same theoretical framework as the study of the person who is using that speech.

An investigation of the relationship between variability in stuttering severity and construing should make it possible to explain one of the overwhelmingly consistent facts about stuttering—that the variability among a group of stutterers may be greater than that *between* groups of stutterers and nonstutterers. Another effect of using a construct theory explanation of stuttering is that it does not lead just to one form of treatment but suggests that changes in construing underlie all responses to therapy, *no matter what form it takes*. The person who responds to the beat of a metronome, a desensitization hierarchy or client-centred therapy, is seen as being one who has been able to take advantage of the situation in which he now finds himself and to reconstrue himself in relation to fluency. If he can build up a system of constructs and implications to make fluency more meaningful, so he will be more likely to gain and maintain that fluency. Such conceptual changes are regarded as the common denominator running through all forms of treatment in which stutterers have improved. Because of its emphasis on reconstruction and on increasing the meaningfulness of being fluent, this therapy goes beyond the point at which most therapies cease. It is only when the stutterer is relatively fluent that he can begin to experiment fully with his new-found way of life. He is seen as needing guidance during this experimental stage. Some of his experiments will be failures and he will need help in construing the invalidating evidence.

IX. A Summary of the Theory

The theoretical position advanced here is that a person stutters because he knows how to do it. He does not have a maladaptive response, a symptom, a disease or a deficiency. To the contrary, he is a success and not a failure, he has an adaptation, a skill. The fluent person cannot stutter nearly so well as the stutterer can because he lacks the years of experience needed. What the stutterer lacks is the skill of fluency.

The stutterer cannot communicate in harmony with fluent people or develop the skill of fluency because no one has told him the rules of the game. Communication between human beings is vastly complex, depending not on the words said, but more on the *way* in which they are spoken, including all the non-verbal cues such as whether one looks the other in the eye or not, types of hand and body gesture, not to mention tone of voice and verbal emphases.

No wonder the stutterer keeps on exercising this skill of his. He knows how to relate to people when he stutters but they are a mystery to him when he does not. The male transvestite could be quite at home playing the part of a woman in both male and female company because he thinks (construes) like a woman and he can interpret the responses of both sexes (although he may be more skilful at communicating with women than with men). However, the normal man would be greatly confused by the reactions of both sexes if he suddenly became, to all outward appearances, a woman.

So the stutterer has to find out what life will all be about when he becomes fluent. The central theme of this theory is that *the road from stuttering to fluency is paved by reconstructions.*

Section III

The Research Project

CHAPTER 5

Measures Used

Not that the scientifically-minded psychologist does not ordinarily try to say simply that A is true; nor does he expect his data to tell him that A is true. Moreover, he does not expect his data to tell him *how much truth* there is in A, as if there could be an absolute measure of the amount of truth inherent in A, independent of its context of B and C. In order to make sense the researcher has to ask *which of two things, in comparison with each other,* is true. Actually his context implies at least three, rather than two, things, but the rest of the like elements in the context can often remain unmentioned. Thus the researcher nowadays usually designs his research around two rival hypotheses and asks the data to tell him *which, in a given sense and in comparison with the other,* is true.

All of this is very much in line with the epistomological position we have called *constructive alternativism.* For we must keep trying our alternative interpretations on nature for size, since she never offers to give us her measurements in advance. Only by comparisons of what we contrive to try on do we successively approximate the one ultimate hypothesis that is truer than any other. It should be clear, then, that what any scientist can hope to discover is not an absolute categorical truth, nor even a relative fraction of truth, but a categorical truth applied in a context of relationships. The relativity refers not to the truth—that is categorical—but to the hypotheses in the context of which truth is the abstraction.

G. A. Kelly (1955)

In modern psychology research and measurement walk hand in hand like two "in-laws" who know they have to get on for the sake of harmony within the family but are not always too happy about the relationship. One of the major problems in the measurement of "personality factors" has focused on what to measure. For construct theory there has been no such problem. The unit of measurement is *the construct*—a way in which two things are alike and thereby different from the third. There are of course innumerable problems associated with the measurement of construct relationships, but at least the unit is defined.

The decision about what, when and how to measure speech disfluencies is also fraught with difficulties. As with construct theory, the unit to be measured can be stated in general terms but when we come to try and define what we mean by *disfluency*, problems start.

Not only is there a problem in defining *what* to measure but account has also to be taken of the fact that a stutterer's speech can be affected by the varied constructions he places on events in his immediate environment. One day may be a "good day"; he wakes up feeling well and, while enjoying this state of well-being, has relatively error-free speech. The next day the reverse may be the case. Also to be considered are such things as the "adaptation effect" (speech errors tend to decrease as the disfluent person becomes "familiar" with a particular situation) and the various speech idiosyncracies of the members of the group being studied.

Research goes on in spite of what, at times, seem like insuperable difficulties. This does not imply a belief in the notion that "if you don't look at them they will go away", only that meaningful results can be obtained but they must be interpreted in the full awareness of some of the other factors that might have influenced them.

The present research was an attempt to investigate the hypothesis that *a stutterer's disfluencies would decrease as meaningfulness of being a fluent speaker increased*. Twenty stutterers were taken on for treatment, conducted along lines dictated by personal construct theory. At intervals each stutterer was given a form of repertory grid, to measure the "meaningfulness" of being fluent, and had samples of reading and spontaneous speech recorded from which measures of disfluencies and speed of speech could be taken. Descriptions of these measures and of the group of stutterers treated will be given followed by details of the results.

I. Measurement of Construing

A. REPERTORY GRID TECHNIQUE

A Description

This technique, described by Kelly to enable one to index the relationships between some of the constructs an individual uses to interpret events in his "world", has evolved into many forms since 1955. However, all forms have certain basic similarities. They are designed to establish the pattern of relationships between constructs for an individual, rather than to compare this patterning to the patternings given by others. There is nothing to prevent one obtaining results from groups and comparing an individual's results with these [e.g. Bannister and Fransella's (1967) Grid Test of Thought Disorder], but the focus of the technique is upon the individual's construing system. All forms of grid are devoid of a fixed form of content—it is a *technique* and not a *test*, and as a technique it can be designed anew for each specific problem. All existing forms are such that statistical tests of significance can be applied to the rankings, sortings or comparisons that each individual has made. This implies the basic assumption that the statistical relationship reflects the psychological relationship between two constructs.

Kelly's original form of grid was the Role Construct Repertory Test or Rep Test. This he designed to provide the clinician with ideas about how the person being investigated had come to be in the fix in which he found himself. The person was asked to name twenty or thirty people he knew who fitted the different role titles provided for him, such as "your boss", "a person you dislike", "a person you admire", and so forth. These Kelly called the *elements* and they form the basis for the elicitation of *constructs*. Constructs are elicited by presenting the person with three of the elements and asking him in what important way two are alike and thereby different from the third. The reply could be that two are *relaxed* people and the person probably indicates to which people he is referring. He is then asked how the third person (element) differs from the other two, and he may answer that he is *tensed up all the time*. This similarity (relaxed) and contrast (tensed up all the time) is a construct dimension. In the Rep Test it was from constructs such as these that the clinician hoped to obtain some insight into the way the patient construed his environment and the people in it.

The Rep Test format then evolved into a grid form, which Kelly referred to as the Repertory Test. In this, the role titles are written along the top of the grid square and personal constructs down the side. The subject is required to put a tick under each of the people (elements) to whom the first pole of the construct applies or to leave the cell blank if the opposite pole of the construct is applicable. An example of this form of

Role Figures

	1	2	3	4	5	6	7	8	9	10	11	12	13	14	15	16	17	18	19	20
nice–dull	×		×		×	×				×				×		×			×	×
witty–solemn		×	×		×		×				×		×	×				×		
shy–extravert	×			×			×			×		×			×		×			
happy–unhappy		×	×			×		×			×		×			×		×	×	×
close–extravagant	×						×		×								×			
mischievous–severe	×			×	×						×			×						
unreliable–reliable		×	×		×		×		×		×									

Fig. 4. A Role Construct Repertory Test with 20 role titles and 8 constructs.

grid is shown in Fig. 4. Kelly devised a non-parametric method of factor analysis which could be applied to the ticks and blanks making up the grid matrix. The statistical factors extracted were regarded as indicating some of the fundamental dimensions along which the person construes his world, always limited of course by the particular constructs and elements forming the particular grid.

In 1959, Bannister showed that meaningless correlations could be produced if the ticks and blanks in a matrix had a lopsided distribution. One could get the situation of a person seeing bow-leggedness and beauty queens as being related constructs if only one of his elements could be described as *bow-legged* and only one other as *like a beauty queen*. Kelly had been well aware of this difficulty, and suggested ways in which lopsided rows could be eliminated. Bannister, however, preferred to modify the technique by getting the subject to provide an equal number of ticks and voids. Some people found this forced division of elements artificial and Bannister (1963) next suggested that the elements could be *ranked* in terms of the constructs.

This rank order form was used in the present study to look at some of the ways in which the stutterers view certain situations and is described in 'repertory grid methodology' (see Chapter 8).

Reliability

One question that is often asked concerns the reliability and validity of this measuring procedure. To what extent would one expect to get the same constructs on a second occasion and to what extent would one get the same implications for these constructs?

Kelly is reported as defining reliability as the measure of a test's insensitivity to change. This was no facetious comment, but a logical deduction from a theory which sees man as a form of motion. Mair (1964) has suggested that instead of expecting a measure to yield near identical scores on *all* occasions, one should substitute the notion of predicting whether there should be stability or change.

There can, of course, be no such thing as *the* reliability of repertory grid technique, since there is no one form of the grid. Indeed, Bannister (1960, 1962) has shown that the reliability correlation co-efficient can be used as a score. Schizophrenic patients who think in a characteristic disordered way relate constructs as if each were a separate dimension. They are also inconsistent when they use these dimensions on a second occasion. This inconsistency (unreliability) has been operationally defined in grid terms and incorporated into a test for discriminating thought-disordered schizophrenics from all other groups (Bannister and Fransella, 1966, 1967). Some so-called "normal" people also seem to use constructs as relatively discrete entities, but they use them consistently. Apart from this use of reliability as the basis for a score, several grid studies involving serial testing have shown a high degree of stability of certain constructs over time (e.g. Fransella and Adams, 1966; Fransella and Joyston-Bechal, 1971) and where movement has occurred it has been predictable (e.g. Fransella and Crisp, 1970).

At the end of a long and detailed discussion of reliability in relation to grid technique Bannister and Mair conclude:

One practical rule must be that if the reliability of a particular grid in a particular context needs to be known, for either theoretical or practical reasons, then it will have to be specifically assessed as part of the experimental venture. It is to be hoped that the day of the comprehensive cookbook of tables of grid reliabilities will never come. Such a volume might help perpetuate the tendency to regard high reliability as an experimental necessity, rather than encourage the view that 'reliability' is, in itself, a target for experimental investigation. (Bannister and Mair, 1968, p. 176.)

Validity

What has been said concerning reliability is equally pertinent to the concept of validity. Studies that are directly or indirectly related to the validity of the grid techniques are unsatisfactory for a number of reasons (detailed in Bannister and Mair, 1968), but examples of the sorts of experiments that have been undertaken will give an idea of their scope.

Investigating the Individuality Corollary of the theory (persons differ from each other in their construction of events), Bonarius (1965) cites a study by Payne (1956) in which subjects were better able to predict their partner's answers on a questionnaire when provided with his own constructs than when provided with constructs used by other people about him. It has also been found that people give a more detailed description of their impression of a fictitious person when his qualities are given in terms of their own personal constructs than when they are given "normative" constructs (Delia *et al.*, 1971). These studies imply that one will, for instance, be more successful in predicting a stutterer's responses or reactions to a situation if one is given some of the constructs the stutterer himself uses to make sense of his world than if one has available only "stereotype" constructs that others use to describe stutterers. Similarly, one has a fuller picture of a person if one is allowed to construe him in one's own terms than if one has to use constructs because they are "average" ways of construing people.

Other studies have shown that, for instance, it is possible to predict certain grid scores from pairs of known and unknown words (Mair, 1966); that attitudes to the experimenter and "need for approval" are related to the ease with which subjects respond to verbal conditioning (Knowles and Purves, 1965); and that it is possible to predict voting behaviour at a general election from "political" and evaluative construct relationships in a grid (Fransella and Bannister, 1967).

A few single case studies (e.g. Salmon, 1963; Fransella and Adams, 1966; Bannister and Mair, 1968) have suggested that construct relationships are meaningfully related to what is known about an individual and that certain predicted relationships occur. Bannister and Mair point out that such studies are based on some very simple-minded assumptions, and that much still needs to be done.

Probably the most useful, if not the most frequent, ventures will be those in which the grid is used with a single patient where the approach has formal coherence, so that predictions are made before test, the lines of treatment appropriate to negation or support of the hypothesis specified before test, and the criteria of successful outcome of these predictions are defined in advance. (Bannister and Mair, 1968, p. 200.)

B. IMPLICATION GRIDS

A Description

The present theory of stuttering leans heavily on the major restatement of some of the theoretical aspects of construct theory proposed by Hinkle in 1965. Particularly relevant is the proposition that constructs are defined by their superordinate and subordinate implications—a construct implies some things and is, in turn, implied by others.

Hinkle elicited "superordinate" constructs by what has come to be described as a "laddering" procedure. When a subordinate construct has been elicited by presenting triads of elements, and its opposite determined, the person is asked by which pole of the construct he would prefer to be described. For instance, at one testing session a stutterer said that two elements were people with *strong personalities* and the other was *weak*. He said, understandably enough, that he would prefer to be a *strong personality*. To encourage him to "climb up" his supposedly hierarchically structured construct system, he was asked *why* he would prefer to be seen as a *strong* rather than as a *weak personality* and he said that people with *strong personalities* were admired and the others were not. *Admired–not admired* is a construct superordinate to *strong personalities– weak personalities*. To the question "why would you prefer to be *admired* than *not admired*", the answer might be "because if you are admired it would show people *respected* you". A further step in the ladder might be that if one is *respected* in life he is more likely to *get his own way*. This procedure of asking "why" can be continued until the person is unable to provide any more constructs. When this happens the whole procedure can be repeated with another subordinate construct.

Hinkle was concerned that the subjects should consider the implications of whole constructs and to obtain this result, he gave these rather complex instructions.

Consider this construct for a moment. Now, if you were to be changed back and forth from one side to the other—that is, if you woke up one morning and realized that you were best described by one side of this construct while the day before you had been best described by the opposite side—if you realized that you were changed in this *one* respect—what other constructs of these nineteen remaining ones would be *likely* to be changed by a change in yourself on this one construct alone? Changing back and forth on just this one construct will *probably cause* you to predictably change back and forth on which other constructs? Remember a change on just this one construct is the cause, while the changes on these other constructs are the effects, implied by the changes from one side to the other on this construct alone. What I'd like to find out, then, is on which of these constructs do you probably expect a change to occur as the *result of knowing* that you have changed from one side to the other on this construct alone. A knowledge of your location on this one construct would probably be used to determine your location on which of these remaining constructs? (Hinkle, 1965, p. 37.)

An implications grid based on Hinkle's method takes the form shown in Fig. 5, in which a cross indicates an implied relationship between the column and row construct.

Constructs

	20	19	18	17	16	15	14	13	12	11	10	9	8	7	6	5	4	3	2	1
1							r	r	×							r	×		r	
2							r	r								r			r	
3				×	×					×				×						
4	×	×	r		×	r	r	r	r	r	×		×	×			r			
5				×			r	r	r			×		×			×	r		
6	×			×	×		×	×	×				×			×				
7	×			r	r		×	×	×				×			r	r		r	
8				r																
9					×	×			×	×								×		
10	×	×		×		r	×	×	×											
11	r	r	r	r	r	r		r	r				×							
12	r	×		×	r	r		r		r						r	r			
13				×	r	r	r		r	r						r	r	r	r	
14		×		×		r	×	×		r						r	r	r	r	
15	×			×	r		r	r	r				×	r		×	r		×	
16	×	×	r	×		r	r	r	r				r	r			r			
17	r	r							r											
18	×	×		×	r		×		r	×							r			
19	r			r					r											
20		r		r					r	r										
	20	19	18	17	16	15	14	13	12	11	10	9	8	7	6	5	4	3	2	1

Constructs (left axis, rows 1–20)

Fig. 5. An implications grid in which a row implication is indicated by an × and a reciprocal implication (where *a* implies *b* and *b* implies *a*) is indicated by an r (from Hinkle, 1965).

A preliminary trial soon showed that these instructions and the whole procedure were too complicated for the average stutterer. This was probably because Hinkle's work had been carried out with a University population and the stutterer sample had a wide range of intellectual ability. A simpler procedure, therefore, had to be adopted. It was also

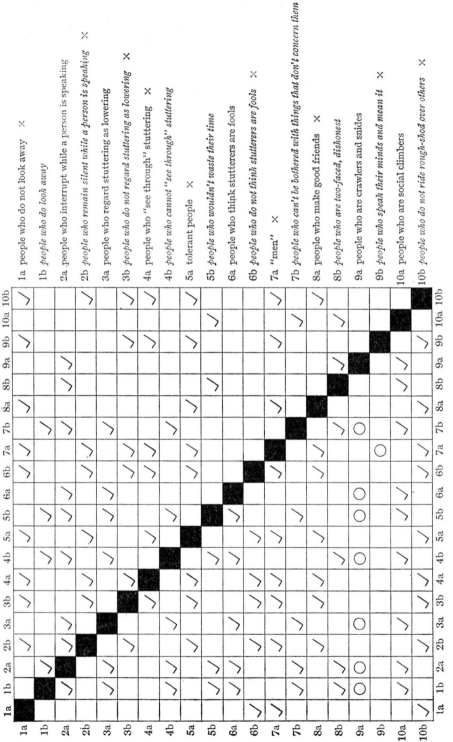

Fig. 6. An example of a bi-polar implications grid. Self-referent construct poles are marked by an X; implicit construct poles are in italics; and the implications of the construct *crawlers and snides/speak their own minds* are shown by circles.

felt that as the emphasis was on the measurement of change, it was important to have an idea of the implications of each pole of a construct. Since an individual is expected to be described by that pole of a construct which is most meaningful to him or "through which he anticipates the greater possibility for increasing the total number of implications in his system", then it would be of use to find out whether there were any constructs on which the person felt himself best described by the pole with the fewer implications.

From time to time an individual may be forced by circumstances, for instance by stuttering, to behave *as if* the opposite pole of a construct applied to him. Part of a bipolar Impgrid of one stutterer in the present sample shows him to have *speaks his mind*, as one pole of a construct. This was both the preferred and self-descriptive pole but it had many fewer implications than its opposite pole, *crawlers and snides*. Figure 6 also shows how a bi-polar Impgrid differs in lay-out from that described by Hinkle (Fig. 5). He could not speak his mind since he is a stutterer and so was forced to behave *as if* he were a *crawler* and a *snide* and had elaborated that pole considerably more than the other.

In order to simplify the procedure and to gain additional information, the Impgrid was modified so that the implications of both poles of each construct could be obtained.

A Bi-Polar Impgrid

The construct theory of stuttering dictated that measures from the Impgrids should be concerned with:

(i) construing of the self in a social context,
(ii) the social construing of individuals and not of groups,
(iii) the relationship between the meaningfulness of being a fluent speaker as opposed to being a stutterer,
(iv) the change in stutterer/fluent speaker meaningfulness over time.

To meet these requirements, the implications grids were constructed so that each person on each test occasion completed two grids based upon two separate sets of elicited constructs, one set to investigate construing of being a stutterer (S-grids) and the other of being a nonstutterer (NS-grids) (Fransella, 1969).

Elicitation. Elicitation of constructs for both grids was based on the construing of four photographs of unknown people of the same sex as the stutterer. Each triad consisted of a pair of photographs *together with* the stutterer himself, represented by a card on which was written *either* ME AS OTHERS SEE ME WHEN I AM *NOT* STUTTERING (for NS-grids) *or* ME AS OTHERS SEE ME WHEN I *AM* STUTTERING (for

S-grids). For each grid there were thus six different triads from which similarities and differences could be construed. The stutterer was asked to think of himself and the two people represented in the photographs as if viewed by a fourth person who might see two of them as being alike in some important way and thereby different from the third. This may sound a difficult task, but very few of the stutterers experienced much trouble after the first pairing, especially as they were given unlimited time to complete the procedure. Only two people had real difficulties, both of lower than average intelligence, one being illiterate with suspected brain damage.

At each presentation the stutterer was allowed to give as many constructs as he liked, but in most cases there was only one obvious way of construing the triad. If he were quite unable to see any way in which two of the three were alike, he was presented with another pair of photographs, the "self" card always remaining present.

Two sets of photographs were used and these were alternated so that on test I if a stutterer completed the first grid with photographs A, at test II he would do the first grid with photographs B.

Laddering. When all six combinations of the photographs had been presented, each construct was "laddered". One of the difficulties encountered during the elicitation of both subordinate and superordinate constructs concerned the procedure for identifying their opposite poles. In practice, one can either ask a person how he would describe the other element(s) in a triad or one can ask what the opposite of the emergent pole is. Laddering presents a similar difficulty. A *strong personality* may be *admired* and the opposite of *admired* may be a person who is *scorned*, but if one were to ladder from both sides of *strong personality–weak personality*, he might find that people who are *weak personalities* are just *ignored*. In the present study the former procedure was adopted—a construct was elicited, from triads or by laddering, and then the opposite asked for. Recent evidence (Epting *et al.*, 1971) suggests that this method gives operationally better opposites than does asking "how does the other person differ". It was found that many stutterers preferred to "ladder" on the non-preferred side, they often would prefer to be 'A' because people who are 'not A' are many things they would not themselves like to be, once again suggesting that this non-preferred side was more meaningful to them.

The Bi-polar Impgrid Format. This format differed from that originally described by Hinkle. As it was deemed necessary to have the implications of each pole separately identified the Impgrid was constructed and administered to each stutterer as follows. Two identical sets of construct cards were prepared—each card having the emergent and implicit pole of a construct written on it, each pole marked 'a' or 'b'. One set of cards (X) was cut in half so that only one pole was on any one card. The set of whole cards (Y) was then laid out in front of the stutterer and the cards in set X were shuffled so that they were in a haphazard order. The stutterer was then presented with one card at a time from set X and told that all he knew about a person was that he was, let us say, *a strong personality*, and was then asked which of the qualities on the cards before him he would *expect* to find in a person with a *strong personality*. He was told to scan the cards before him and when he came across something that was *implied by* being a *strong personality*, he was to read out the number on the card, stating whether it was 'a' or 'b'. A complete bi-polar Impgrid is given in Fig. 7.

In all, ninety-three grids were completed, the maximum completed by any one stutterer being ten, the minimum two.

Unfortunately for scientific purity, the two grids (S and NS) and the speech recordings were not able to be completed on the same day. In fact, the implications grid administration sometimes extended over several sessions. They are extremely time-consuming. This would be a grave disadvantage if these were standardized tests, but they are not. They sometimes even played a part in the reconstruction process itself. Clear evidence of this was given by one man at the second or third testing. While poring over the cards, he suddenly smiled broadly to himself and, after a pause, said "I thought it was only the psychologist who was supposed to learn from the test, not the patient himself!" While doing the grid he had suddenly seen some relationship or implication between constructs of which he had previously been unaware. He never did disclose what it was that had gone through his mind, never stated it overtly that is.

A method of analysis was worked out to show the relationships between the poles of the constructs used (the details of this are given in Appendix I). This statistical procedure for assessing the probabilities of the presence of matching or mis-matching ticks between any two lines was used on the Impgrid in Fig. 7 and some of the statistically significant relationships are shown in Fig. 8.

A procedure for grouping these significant relationships into their main dimensions of construing has yet to be devised, so at the present time it is only meaningful to plot a few in order to give a pictorial representation. Those that are shown are sufficient to indicate the degree to which this young man identified himself with *stutterers* as a group, who had most of the "good" qualities, and how he saw *fluent speakers* as unlike himself and as having most of the "bad" qualities. These results prompted probing into his reasons for seeking treatment. He said (enthusiastically) that he

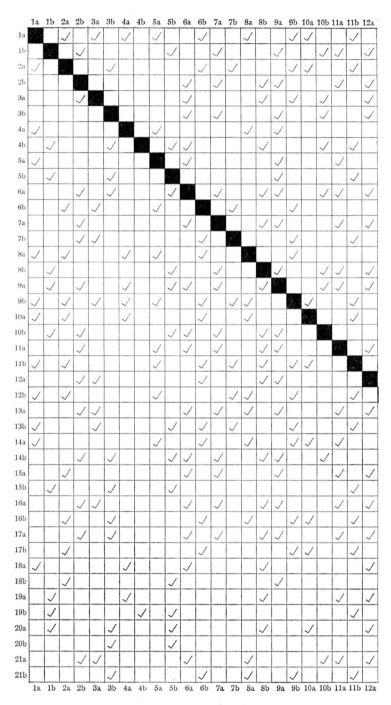

FIG. 7.   Bi-polar implications grid on which was based

12b	13a	13b	14a	14b	15a	15b	16a	16b	17a	17b	18a	18b	19a	19b	20a	20b	21a	21b	
✓			✓						✓		✓								1a ambitious for money or status
	✓		✓																1b *not primarily concerned with money or status*
✓	✓						✓											✓	2a don't consider others at all
	✓				✓														2b *considerate*
	✓			✓	✓				✓										3a hide their feelings
			✓	✓	✓		✓		✓				✓		✓				3b *show their feelings*
			✓	✓							✓								4a "game"
✓			✓		✓				✓		✓	✓							4b accept defeat
	✓	✓						✓							✓				5a like to impress
✓	✓				✓			✓	✓		✓				✓				5b *content with how they appear to others*
	✓		✓					✓	✓				✓						6a *more sensitive*
✓	✓							✓	✓						✓				6b less sensitive
	✓		✓			✓		✓											7a *concerned with small points about others*
✓	✓	✓							✓										7b tied up with themselves
✓							✓		✓		✓								8a forceful
	✓					✓								✓					8b *not forceful*
	✓		✓	✓				✓			✓		✓						9a like me in character (supplied construct)
✓	✓	✓					✓		✓		✓								9b not like me in character (supplied construct)
✓	✓		✓				✓		✓		✓								10a ruthless
			✓			✓		✓	✓										10b *not ruthless*
✓							✓		✓		✓								11a *like to be liked*
✓	✓						✓		✓										11b do not care if liked or not
■	✓		✓	✓					✓						✓		✓		12a *want to avoid embarrassment*
	✓	✓			✓		✓		✓		✓				✓		✓		12b rarely feel embarrassed
	■				✓														13a *do all they can to make social relationships easy*
✓		■	✓	✓		✓		✓										✓	13b don't care if social relationships are easy or not
✓			■								✓								14a respected for material things
✓				■				✓											14b *respected as a person*
✓					■			✓	✓				✓						15a have control over themselves, analyse things
✓			✓			■		✓							✓				15b *open about everything*
	✓						■		✓							✓			16a *don't cause embarrassment*
✓			✓					■	✓						✓		✓	✓	16b cause embarrassment
	✓								■		✓	✓							17a *worry about minor things*
✓	✓					✓				■									17b do not worry about things
✓					✓	✓	✓				■	✓		✓	✓		✓		18a *get irritable and depressed*
												■							18b do not get irritable and depressed
	✓		✓	✓					✓	✓			■	✓					19a *live and plan for the future*
		✓	✓						✓					■					19b live in the present
				✓			✓								■			✓	20a can be caught off guard
																■			20b *never caught off guard*
	✓		✓				✓		✓				✓				■		21a stutterers (supplied construct)
	✓				✓	✓	✓											■	21b nonstutterers (supplied construct)

the plot of significant relationships shown in Fig. 8.

had been persuaded by others and that he did not find his stutter trouble-some at all. He was glad to be given the opportunity to escape treatment. This young man did not form part of the research sample and so there was no problem (from the research point of view) in allowing him to opt out.

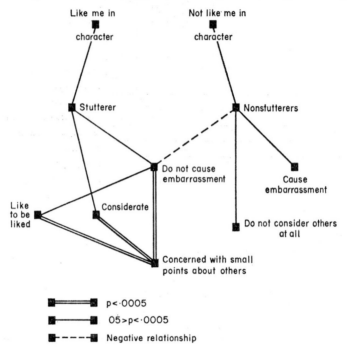

FIG. 8. Pictorial representation of a few of the statistically significant relationships between constructs in a bi-polar implications grid of one stutterer.

C. SELF CHARACTERIZATION

There are many ways of asking questions and the self characterization was one Kelly used to implement his first principle, central to his thinking although never stated formally. It came out something like "if you don't know what's wrong with a person, ask him, he *may* tell you". Kelly did not mean he would tell you in so many words, but his answer might be contained in what he said if one listened carefully enough.

What Kelly did was to ask the person to write a profile of himself on the basis of the following very carefully thought out instructions, with the person's own name substituted for 'Harry Brown':

I want you to write a character sketch of Harry Brown, just as if he were the principal character in a play. Write as it might be written by a friend who knew him very *intimately* and very *sympathetically*, perhaps better than anyone ever really could know him. Be sure to write it in the third person. For example, start out by saying 'Harry Brown is . . .' (Kelly, 1955.)

Kelly had two main reasons for wording the instructions in this particular way. One was to impose a certain amount of structure on the writing so that the person did not provide one with his construct system to do with, say, merely eating habits. The other was to minimize threat by making the description "indirect". Some people feel vulnerable if they put their failings onto paper for all to see, afraid perhaps that they may be laughed at or become the object of sympathy.

Almost without exception, the present group of stutterers reported that this was a difficult task, but that they had found it very interesting and, in some cases, very illuminating. No attempt has been made to analyse these protocols in any formal way, although Kelly does suggest how this might be done (1955, p. 319). Their purpose in the research was two-fold. The self characterization provides an additional source of information for the therapist about the ways a person is viewing his world. Also, by writing a self characterization from time to time, the person is encouraged to verbalize changes, if any, that may have occurred in his way of looking at life. Extracts from some self characterizations will be found in the next chapter, where a brief account is given of each stutterer treated.

II. Measurement of Disfluencies

A. problems of measurement

There are at least four factors that have to be considered when attempting to measure changes in stuttering behaviour.

(i) when should one take the measures,
(ii) how should one deal with the adaptation that may occur during repeated measurement,
(iii) what is to be considered as improvement,
(iv) what is one going to measure.

When to Measure

Milisen (1957) has concluded that the quantification of a stutterer's speech "need not involve highly accurate measurement of overt symptoms or attitudes, because the conditions change so markedly from one period to another and from one situation to another". Quarrington (1965) points out that there are overall day to day fluctuations in severity of stuttering as well as in the specific situations that are likely to evoke either severe stuttering or virtually non-existent stuttering. Sheehan

(1969) cites some evidence of Quarrington showing significant cyclic variation ranging from two to six months in 59% of a group of four-year-old children who were rated by their mothers over a period of one year. Systematic fluctuation also occurred in the ratings of the stutterer reported here in detail and discussed in Chapter 9.

There seems no really satisfactory way in research for dealing with the day to day variability of speech for any individual. Thus, testing times were decided upon before the client turned up for his appointment, and went ahead irrespective of whether it turned out to be a "good" or a "bad" day. In this way it was possible, hopefully, to even out the effect of variability in speech. The testing situation was varied in terms of place and person doing the testing so that the total situation was considered to be one liable to elicit maximal disfluency. Whether the aim was successful or not, there is no way of knowing.

The Adaptation Effect

There is no doubt at all that stuttering decreases if the same passage of prose or list of words is read a number of times when there is little or no interval between the readings, as well as when the person is speaking spontaoeously. But the presence and degree of adaptation is determined by many factors and there is now an extensive literature on the subject (see Beech and Fransella, 1968). Apart from situational adaptation, Trotter and Kools (1955) point out the importance of the adaptation of the *listener* in rating speech severity. Therapists may well rate their clients as having improved because they have adapted to the stutterer's speech defect over time—they have got used to it.

Johnson (1955) considered the lawfulness of this effect as a "laboratory model of the improvement process" and in 1965 Lanyon tested this idea experimentally. He correlated the degree of adaptation at the start of the year's treatment programme for thirty-three stutterers with change in rate of utterance, total number of disfluencies and ratings of severity. Although the correlation between the measure of adaptation and clinician's rating and speaking rate were statistically significant (0·36 and 0·34 respectively), he concluded that the correlations were too small to be of any clinical importance. He may be understating the case as Prins (1968) reported results showing adaptation to be *negatively* related to amount of change in disfluencies after treatment.

Because of the variability of stuttering and, to date, the lack of success in demonstrating anything approaching a close relationship between degree of adaptation and likelihood of improvement, no attempt was made to examine this possible prognostic indicator in the present study. However, the experimental design ensured, as far as possible, that the therapist did the minimum of testings after the initial session. Out of the fifty-two speech test occasions, twenty-eight were carried out by the author (twenty being first testings) and twenty-four by other personnel.

What Is Improvement?

Of more practical importance perhaps is the question "when is a stutterer no longer a stutterer"? Presumably when neither he nor his listeners call him one. Many experts have stated that they do not believe that there is any such thing as "cured" stutterers. However free from "stutter-type" disfluencies they are, given the right environmental situation, with appropriate stresses and strains, they will revert to their previous well-established speech pattern, even if it is only for a very short space of time. This is hardly surprising considering that someone of thirty years of age may well have been using a stuttering speech pattern for twenty-five years of his life and his "fluent" pattern for only one year. So while total elimination of stuttering and increased rate of speech must be the ultimate aim, this may hardly ever be realized.

For the majority of stutterers "improvement" is relative and can normally be considered to consist of an *increase* in rate of speaking or reading and a *decrease* in disfluencies. But this is not an infallible rule. Among the twenty stutterers treated in this research, the aims for two were in the opposite direction (excluding the man diagnosed as a clutterer—one in whom an excessive rate of speaking is a prominent feature). One was a girl who had what can only be described as "an excessive flow of words". She had no fluency problems in general conversation at a speed of around 234 words per minute but in situations in which she was anxious, as over the telephone, she attempted to maintain this rate and stuttered severely, often blocking completely. One of the aims in her case, therefore, was to get her to reduce rather than increase her speed of speaking. The other instance of a reversal of aims was of the man who had so perfected an avoidance technique that no semblance of a stutter was apparent in his general conversation. He could "see" words coming along on which he expected trouble and was able to select an alternative "non-troublesome" word; all this he achieved while speaking at around 136 words per minute. However, in his work as a journalist he was required to read such things as the winners of a race over the telephone. In such a situation he was unable to "avoid" and his stutter became apparent. Thus, the aim for him was, initially at least, to encourage him to increase rather than to decrease his disfluencies.

Apart from these two stutterers, improvement was considered significant if there was a reduction in disfluencies of more than 50%.

What to Measure?

The lack of agreement as to the definition and hence diagnosis of what everyone recognizes as stuttering has already been discussed in Chapter I. Although Johnson has shown that there is considerable overlap between the nonstutterer with a number of disfluencies and the stutterer with only a few, these disfluencies do seem to be of a different type. For instance, listeners seem to be significantly influenced by the presence of single-unit and double-unit syllable repetitions (ma-marmalade; ma-ma-marmalade) and sound prolongations. Thus any measure of disfluencies should include these.

Wendahl and Cole (1961) found that listeners were able to distinguish between recorded speech samples of stutterers and nonstutterers even when the actual disfluencies had been eliminated. Apparently the listeners were basing their decisions on the slower rate of speaking, the greater force used and the general lack of rhythm in the speech. General flow and force of speech would be hard to quantify without using a number of raters but increased rate of speech can be taken as a measure.

The methods of speech analysis used attempted to take all four factors into account as far as possible.

B. METHODS OF ANALYSIS

Disfluency Measures

Johnson and others (1963) advocate the use of eight categories of disfluency: interjections of sounds, syllables, words or phrases; part-word repetitions; word repetitions; phrase repetitions; revisions; incomplete phrases; broken words and prolonged sounds. Young (1961) found that the sum of part-word repetitions, prolonged sounds, broken words and words unusually stressed, correlated 0·85 with rated severity. He therefore suggested the use of a single category of "repetitions" as an operational definition of disfluency. At the same time Sander (1961) was advocating the use of a very similar overall category of "disfluent" words (i.e. words including prolonged sounds; broken words; sound, syllable or word repetitions; words interrupted by interjections). He found that his disfluent word count correlated 0·87 for speaking and 0·86 for reading, with a sum total of Johnson's disfluencies. Apart from Johnson using more categories of disfluencies, the measures differ in that for total disfluencies every one occurring is counted, whereas a disfluent word is only counted once no matter how many disfluences occur on it.

In view of these studies it was decided to use measures of both total disfluencies and Sander's disfluent words since, although the correlations between these measures are high, 15–17% of the variance is still un-accounted for. Any difference obtained between these two methods of scoring adds to the description of an individual's overall stuttering pattern. For instance, a person can be disfluent a large number of times in just a few words giving a high total disfluency, and a low disfluent word score or he can have just one disfluency on many words giving a low total disfluency and high disfluent word score.

Sander's reported correlations between reading and speaking were 0·72 for total disfluencies and 0·70 for disfluent words, indicating that the use of both reading and speaking samples might also provide additional information. Rate of reading was found to correlate above 0·80 with both measures of disfluency but, again, a considerable amount of vari-ance was unaccounted for.

In the light of this information counts of total disfluencies and dis-fluent words plus rate of utterance were based on tape-recorded speech samples. On each test occasion the speech samples consisted of two-minutes of spontaneous speech and the reading of a passage of prose. The spontaneous speech was for the most part a description of the stutterer's present work situation. The reading matter consisted of one of two passages, equated for difficulty by Krikler (unpublished manuscript).

The interval between tests was at least six weeks. There is no convinc-ing evidence that the adaptation effect is operative over as long an inter-val as twelve weeks so, if the stutterer was tested more than twice, the reading passages were used again. Speaking and reading tests were also systematically alternated. Thus, the first person spoke first and then read from Passage I on the first test occasion and read Passage 2 first and spoke second, on the second test occasion. Collecting speech samples in this way and using tape-recordings, was expected to maximize stuttering in all subjects. All speech samples were scored at the completion of the research.

Twenty samples of speaking were randomly selected for re-analysing at an interval of one to two weeks; the test–retest correlation for total disfluencies was 0·92. In all comparisons Spearman rho correlations have been used because of the lack of information concerning equality of intervals in the measures.

Rating Scales

Objective rating scales of severity were not used because, after re-viewing the literature, Beech and Fransella (1968) concluded that to obtain a high reliability of rating, each rating should be done more than once or more than one judge should rate each speech sample. Since this author could not do the rating, because of the possibility of being influenced by her knowledge of the patient and the hypothesis, this would have involved the expenditure of an excessive amount of time on the part of a third party.

However, two types of rating of stuttering severity other than scales were used. One was a subjective assessment by each stutterer of his speech. Johnson *et al.*, (1963) advocated that the stutterer should rate himself on the severity of his stuttering. Beech and Fransella (1968) point out that this presents the interesting problem of the standard against which the self-assessment is made. As the stutterer's speech changes, so his "standard" may change. What was "good" some time ago may well be "bad" after some improvement has taken place. However, these self assessments are important, since it is very relevant to the stutterer's whole progress and state in the situation that he and the therapist know how *he* assesses himself.

Thus, each stutterer was required to rate the severity of speech during the interval since his last visit. He had to rate *average* severity of his speech problem, the *best* it had been and the *worst* on a 7-point scale ranging from "1", indicating best imaginable, to "7", being worst imaginable. It was emphasized that he was to rate how he *felt* his speech had been, and was not to attempt to relate this to some external criteria, such as his girl friend's opinion.

Unfortunately, these self ratings were not always recorded in a systematic way as they were considered to be important in the therapeutic situation rather than as research data. An analysis of one case in which they were taken every session shows this to have been a mistake.

The second rating procedure was used for purely descriptive purposes. The Andrews-Harris Scale of severity of stuttering (1964) categorizes the stutter according to the percentage of disfluent words, as indicated below.

Grade 0: Stammer not heard at interview

Grade 1: Mild Stammer
   Communication unimpaired
   0–5% of words stammered

Grade 2: Moderate stammer
   Communication slightly impaired
   6–20% of words stammered

Grade 3: Severe stammer
   Communication definitely impaired
   Over 20% of words stammered

C. SUMMARY

Twenty stutterers completed "stutterer" (S) and "non-stutterer" (NS) implications grids to measure changes in attitudes to their speech together with self characterizations at intervals during treatment. Two measures of disfluency and rate of utterance were taken from a series of recordings of reading and spontaneous speech. The Andrews-Harris rating scale was used for descriptive purposes only and some stutterers rated their own speech prior to the therapeutic session, but these were not recorded systematically.

CHAPTER 6

The Sample

What for the nomothetist is hard to contemplate is the very real possibility that no two lives are alike in their motivational processes.
Liberalism and the Motives of Men. Frontiers of Democracy
G. W. Allport (1940)

I. GROUP DETAILS

The sample consisted of twenty adults, seventeen men and three women, who were referred to St. George's Hospital, London, for treatment of stuttering. The selection criteria were that they should (a) be over seventeen years of age; (b) have no demonstrable psychiatric disorder or psychiatric history; and (c) have stuttered as long as they could remember. The first twenty stutterers satisfying these criteria were taken on for treatment in the order in which they were referred.

Each stutterer completed a personality questionnaire (the Eysenck Personality Inventory), giving measures of "extraversion–introversion" and "neuroticism", and an intelligence test (the AH4), giving "verbal" and "performance" scores. Table I gives the means and standard deviations on these tests, together with ages, for the group together with normative data for nonstutterers where these are available. The lie scores (L-score) on the Eysenck test were calculated but no inferences were made about individuals since no data were available at the time of the research with which they could be compared. The scores on these tests reported in the following descriptions of each individual stutterer forming the sample, can be compared with the average for his group and with that for the general population. The intercorrelations show that only one of these personality or intelligence measures was significantly related to any of the speech or conceptual measures. This was between the AH4 total intelligence score and nonstutterer implications. The psychological significance of this relationship is discussed in Chapter 7, p. 119. There was no significant difference between the verbal and performance scores on the intelligence test.

Self characterizations were written by the stutterers at intervals during their treatment, roughly coinciding with the testing occasions. These self characterizations can be very revealing and therefore only those parts which refer directly to the stutterer's attitude to his speech are reported

94

verbatim, unless permission has been given by the person concerned for other extracts to be published. In the following descriptions pseudonyms are used throughout.

II. THE INDIVIDUALS

A. WILLIAM

At the start of treatment this man was twenty-one years old, and worked as a computer operator. He believed he started stuttering at about the age of five, and remembered having speech therapy when he was about fourteen which resulted in some improvement. He knew of no family history of stuttering and he was right-handed. He attended the hospital eighty-two times in all (his last few appointments were at two-monthly intervals) and during this period he married, and was promoted in his job three times. He considered that the improvement in his speech greatly helped in these promotions.

TABLE I

Means, standard deviations and ranges of age, scores on the AH4 intelligence test and the Eysenck Personality Inventory for the group of twenty stutterers and the general population.

	Mean	Stutterers S.D.	Range	General Population Mean	S.D.
Age	26·2	8·1	18–50	—	—
AH4 Verbal Score	37·2	9·9	14–56	—	—
AH4 Performance Score	43·1	7·3	26–52	—	—
AH4 Total Score	79·37	15·62	40–108	47·17	19·37
EPI, N Score	10·2	5·6	1–20	9·07	4·78
EPI, E Score	10·3	3·8	1–16	12·07	4·37
EPI, L Score	2·78	1·25	1–5	—	—

His speech defect consisted mainly of part-word repetitions and of broken words (i.e. *guh-guh-girl* and *be*-(pause)*lief*, respectively). On the Andrews-Harris Scale of Severity (see p. 92) he was Grade 2 (Moderate) at the start and Grade 1 (Mild) at the end of treatment. There was, in fact, so little of his speech defect apparent at the last testing that he was judged to have reduced his disfluent words and total disfluencies by over 90%. His scores on the Eysenck Personality Inventory were 8 on neuroticism (N-score) and 3 on extraversion (E-score) and on the AH4 his verbal and performance scores were 39, giving him a total score of 78.

Extracts from two self characterizations

(a) (at the start of treatment)

... He feels he does not really need other people in his life except one or two close friends, and likes to think that he would be completely happy on his own. However, he has a sneaking feeling that if he was alone he would be lonely, and therefore continues to maintain his circle of friends and acquaintances.

He attempted to analyse himself about his attitude towards other people. He felt that just once or twice he would like to break out and be an extrovert personality—the life and soul of the party. Then he realizes that this would be a complete break of character and he would only feel a fool doing it. He appreciates that he is a quiet character; other people realize this, and either like or dislike him for what he is, and not for what he appears to be. Perhaps he feels that by being a livelier person he would be appreciated more by the people he likes; conversely he feels that he is quite well liked as he is, and needs nothing further.

He has wondered whether having a stammer has brought about this feeling of not really needing the majority of other people, or even vice versa, though his defect does not greatly influence his relationships with people he is in everyday contact with, but it is certainly an obstacle with strange people.

(b) (two years later)

... Insofar as other people are concerned, he can't seem to make up his mind whether he cares what other people think of him or not. He would like to be one of those people who go their own way through life, but in practice he generally likes to get on well with most people.

He thinks of himself as being pretty ordinary insofar as relationships with other people are concerned. He tends to adopt a chameleon-like method of conversation to suit the person to whom he is speaking, and now that his stammer has diminished this applies to both delivery and content. He believes himself to be a rather dull conversationalist; previously his conversation was limited by his stammer, but now he thinks the reason is shyness. In his case shyness constitutes his taking care not to be put into a situation where he is likely to be embarrassed, and his conversation tends to be rather conservative. After knowing people for some time however, he reasons that they know enough about him anyway, and he becomes a little more forthcoming.

Now that his stammer has become infrequent, he believes that he cannot now be classified as a "stammerer" but can be accepted for what he is.

Follow-up

Nineteen months after the end of treatment he rated himself as "very much better" and reported his speech to be fairly stable. The steady improvement he had experienced during the treatment period had clearly continued afterwards.

B. MARY

This twenty-five year old woman was a graduate research worker. She believed she started stuttering at the age of five and had been treated on several previous occasions, both at school and after, by speech therapy and by hypnosis. She felt that none of the treatments had produced any demonstrable effect. She was aware of no family history of stuttering and was left-handed. She attended for forty-eight sessions excluding follow-up interviews and during that time obtained her Ph.D. degree and got married.

Her speech was rated as Grade 2 (Moderate) both at the start and at the end of treatment on the Andrews-Harris Severity Scale. But, in fact, there was a 54% reduction in total speech disfluencies.

Her speech defect was characterized by severe blocking, resulting in her making straining noises in her effort to get the words out. Most distressing, both for her and for the onlooker, was the involuntary thrusting out of her tongue which occurred during speech. This involuntary tongue-thrusting totally disappeared and follow-up eighteen months later showed no reappearance of this distressing action, although there had been some fluctuations in the stutter which she related to certain personal difficulties. By the end of treatment she was stuttering less on fewer words and had ceased to thrust out her tongue.

Her scores on the Eysenck Personality Inventory were 6 on neuroticism and 1 on extraversion, and on the AH4 she obtained a verbal score of 43 and a performance score of 44 giving a total score of 87.

Extracts from two self characterizations

(a) (at the start of treatment)

> . . . She is wary and suspicious in relationships with other people. This merges with an inability to say what she wants and in the tone required. Depending on her mood, she tends to fear being misunderstood and avoids speaking to people, or will go ahead and in desperation is often rather rude. Basically she wants to mix easily with people but seems unable to do so. She has always found it difficult to suffer fools gladly and equally difficult to conceal her exasperation . . .

(b) (two years later)

> . . . She is adaptable to the environment and feels she can settle almost anywhere but is too easily influenced by other people's moods and attitudes . . . She does not like crowds, parties or cities for more than a short time but has no desire to become a hermit . . .

Follow-up

Two years after the cessation of treatment, Mary reported that her speech had continued to improve, although it still gives her some trouble particularly when she is tired or ill.

C. GEOFFREY

This twenty-one year old Nigerian was a student at a Technical College. He had stuttered as long as he could remember, and reported having had no previous treatment. He was not aware of any family history and he was right-handed. The nearest he got to receiving treatment prior to his being referred to St. George's Hospital, was from his General Practitioner in Nigeria. This doctor told him to buy records and sing to them, since Geoffrey had commented that he did not stutter when singing. However, when there was no improvement to this "singing" therapy he was given Librium, but again there was no change. He had been in England eight months before seeking further help. He had learned English at school but this was not his first language.

He was accepted for treatment with some reservation since, in addition to his stammer, his English was very difficult to understand. As the whole essence of the approach is to attempt to understand the construing system used by the stutterer, it seemed that difficulty in understanding what was being said might prove an insuperable problem. However, this proved to be of no importance at all; at time of discharge he was virtually fluent.

He attended for twenty-one sessions and no follow-up was possible as he is believed to have returned to Nigeria. His speech defect was mainly characterized by word repetitions and sound prolongations and was rated as Grade 2 (moderate) at the start and Grade 1 (zero disfluent words) at the end of treatment. His scores on the Eysenck Personality Inventory were 14 on neuroticism and 12 on extraversion on the AH4 his verbal and performance scores were 36 giving a total score of 72.

The change in speech was not gradual as with the majority of stutterers referred, but occurred dramatically over a two-week period. It was suggested to him that his problem in speaking to his father and other authority figures could be the result of maintaining a childhood way of construing *senior people* as being *superior people*—his father had always been very severe with him. His father was due to visit this country from Nigeria the following week, and Geoffrey suddenly announced that he was convinced he would no longer have any trouble with speaking to his father since he would see him as his *junior*! He was utterly convinced that this new way of construing his father would work. It did. The following week his stutter was virtually non-existent and he reported that he had been fluent with his father for the first time in his life and that his father had been delighted. It was, however, suggested to him that it might be more realistic to see people as *equals* rather than as *juniors* or *inferiors*. He kept two further appointments, at monthly intervals, during which time he had maintained the improvement.

Follow-up

Contact was lost with this young man so no follow-up was possible.

D. JOHN

This thirty-eight year old man was a chartered engineer. He believed he started stuttering at five or six years of age. He was aware of no family history and was right-handed. Included among his many previous attempts at treatment were (a) having his tonsils out as a child; (b) speech therapy in his teens using a "shadowing" technique, which he said had no effect at all; (c) hypnosis for two years, which had an immediate but not a long-term effect; (d) a repeat of hypnosis—again with no long-term effect; (e) returned to an earlier speech therapist with no effect; (f) further hypnosis after hearing a lecture, which again produced an immediate good effect but not a long-term one.

On the Andrews-Harris Severity measure his speech was Grade 2 (Moderate) at the start of treatment, changing to Grade 1 (Mild) at the last testing after having attended twenty-three times. His speech defect was characterized by blocks, accompanied by general muscle tension and a sudden jerk of the neck or arm, which originally was used to release the spasm. His scores on the EPI were neuroticism 15 and extraversion 12 and on the AH4 he had a verbal score of 30 and a performance score of 43 giving a total score of 73.

Unlike the majority of the sample, this man had most difficulty with his speech at home, particularly when he was trying to explain something complicated to his wife. He was apparently also bad when talking with his children. Due to changes in his place of work, the course of treatment was bedevilled by cancellations. These were usually made by his wife over the telephone, except on one occasion when his wife wrote a letter. After one cancellation and change of place of working he failed to keep any further appointments and all attempts to arrange a follow-up appointment or obtain some indication of his present level of stuttering have failed. Although there was a reduction of 43·3% in total disfluencies and 80% in disfluent words over this erratic treatment period, it seems very unlikely that this improvement was maintained, in view of the short-lasting benefits derived from other treatments. However, it was felt that the prognosis was good if he could have been persuaded to continue treatment since some reconstruing was apparent.

In cases such as this it would have been of advantage to see husband and wife together, since it seemed that the marital role relationships were intimately connected with John's stuttering severity. In view of the wife's role in the making and breaking of appointments it seems likely that she was an important factor in the maintenance of her husband's speech defect. Perhaps she needed him to depend on her for some psychological reason. But it was felt that the research programme as laid down could not include such a procedure.

E. SUSAN

This twenty year old girl was a typist, was not aware of any family history and was right-handed. Her mother came with her on the first occasion and seemed to be more concerned about her daughter's speech than was the girl herself. Her speech was indeed very rapid, but she had few disfluencies when speaking spontaneously. However, when reading or talking on the telephone the blocks and repetitions were severe. Her rate of reading at the first testing was only 37·8 words per minute (average for female nonstutterers being around 177). She thought she had had difficulty since starting to speak, and received speech therapy at school. As was the case with John, she was unusual in this sample in reporting that her speech was at its worst at home. It was likely that there was some relationship between this and the fact that her mother was also an extremely rapid speaker. The girl herself explained her rapid speech as a feeling that she must talk as fast as possible so as to minimize the risk of blocking—a feeling not at all uncommon in stutterers.

The aim of treatment for this girl was therefore two-fold; first to reduce her speed of speaking, and second to help her in specific situations such as telephoning, reading and to stop her feeling she must, for instance, have the right money on the bus or in a shop to reduce the likelihood of her having to speak. The degree to which this was successful is not indicated by the rated severity on the Andrews-Harris scale as it was Grade 1 (Mild) at the start of treatment. She had, in fact, increased her rate of reading and decreased her rate of speaking and had no disfluent words on either speech sample at the end of treatment, seventeen sessions later. She broke off treatment, prior to getting married, since she was moving some way out of London. Her scores on the EPI were 1 on neuroticism and 15 on extraversion. On the AH4 she had a verbal score of 29 and a performance score of 41 giving a total score of 70.

Follow-up

Unfortunately she did not respond to any requests for follow-up appointments.

F. MICHAEL

This twenty-four year old man was single and worked in an office where he found his stutter a problem when telephoning. There was a family history of stuttering—his father's twin brother. He was right-handed.

He had received some speech therapy at school but had not tried any other form of treatment since then. His defect was rated Grade 2 (Moderate) at the start, improving to Grade 1 (Mild) at the end of treatment, and it consisted very largely of syllable repetitions. At the end of eight months, during which he attended nineteen times, he reported that he was not aware of any speech problem at all and made no attempt to "avoid" words. On the EPI he had a neuroticism score of 6 and an extraversion score of 14. On the AH4 he had a verbal score of 38 and a performance score of 46 giving a total score of 84.

Extracts from self characterizations

(a) (at the start of treatment)

> . . . is a fairly shy and reserved person, but he is a reliable friend and hardworking . . . he worries that other people will think it funny when he stutters and will make fun . . . his work would improve if only he could speak out and give orders—show his authority—but here his speech does hold him back . . . It is a pity that he is always thinking about his speech, but it seems to be on his mind all the time, and I feel that his general knowledge is very good and therefore he should be able to hold conversations with friends old and new.

(b) (towards the end of treatment)

> . . . appears to have suddenly become very talkative . . . he seems to be able now to stand and carry on a conversation with total strangers. At work he is giving instructions and orders over the phone with ease, stumbling occasionally when he is a bit harassed, but that happens to us all at times. Even his boss and staff have noticed that he is pushing himself to the front, which is about time. His sudden increase in reading seems to be opening him up a lot more, finding subjects which he knows about therefore finding it easier to talk about them to other people.

Follow-up

A comment from a follow-up letter after nine months was "generally speaking my speech has improved 100-fold—in fact until you wrote I had not given it much thought. I have asked everyone with whom I come in contact every day and the general view is a vast improvement since I last saw you, especially on the telephone. Myself, I cannot remember the last time I was bad on the telephone."

G. HENRY

This twenty year old Malaysian was studying law at university. He started stuttering at the age of six, after a tonsil operation, and has stuttered ever since. His speech was worse in his own language than in

English, which he started speaking at the age of five and did not regard as his "first" language. His speech had shown some improvement two years previously but stuttering became severe again after he failed an examination. He was aware of no family history and reported that he had a tendency to write with his left hand when at school, but was forced to write with his right hand, although his parents requested his teacher not to do this.

He reported that his worst speech was usually with his father and best with his mother. His speech was rated Grade 1 (Mild) at both the start and end of treatment and consisted mainly of blocks which were followed by interjections. This lack of change in grade again masks the fact that during the twenty occasions on which he attended for treatment, his speech improved steadily both in his view and in measured terms, there being an 81% reduction in disfluent words. His scores on the EPI were 17 for neuroticism and 12 for extraversion. On the AH4 he had a verbal score of 49 and a performance score of 47 giving a total score of 96.

Extract from self characterization

(a) (at start of treatment)

> . . . He has grown to believe that his stammer was a social taboo. He keeps away from company and when he's in company he keeps silent unless it's essential to speak. Emotionally he is at a low ebb and is very sensitive to what- ever is said or done to him. He keeps his worries to himself; his stammer re- appears in leaps and bounds when he has something on his mind.

Follow-up

He did not return for any further treatment after his sessional exami- nations, which he had already failed once, and there was no reply to any request for a follow-up appointment. It seems fairly probable that he had failed his examinations a second time and so had returned home to Malaysia.

H. ANDREW

This young man of twenty-three was referred from the dental depart- ment of a London hospital to the speech therapy department and from there to St. George's Hospital. Previous treatments had included hypnosis and attendance at a speech training school where he was given "tongue-twisters"; he believed it was these that have caused his present severe stutter. On the Measure of Severity his speech was rated Grade 2 (Moderate) both at the start of treatment and at the end of treatment. The decrease of 34% in total disfluencies and an increase of 11% in dis- fluent words indicates that, during treatment, he came to stutter less on any one word but was disfluent on slightly more words.

His defect was indeed grotesque to observe. He would be talking quite normally when suddenly his jaw would go rigid, fall half open, and his tongue protrude; his breathing would become violent as he tried to break the spasm, and this would make him dribble and spray saliva as long as the contortion lasted. Sometimes his jaw would just open and shut violently with the muscles seemingly being in spasm. In addition to these very severe accompanying motor disturbances, he was found to have a reading and spelling age of just over 7 years. Because of the reading disability he was given the Progressive Matrices Intelligence Test instead of the AH4 and this gave him an IQ equivalent of 80. He had been regarded as of 'border-line' intelligence at school, and was also thought to have suffered some brain-damage at birth. His General Practitioner thought there might have been some additional brain damage as the result of an accident two years previously, and it was this that was considered to be the cause of his stutter becoming worse.

He was unable to complete the Implications Grids as he seemed not to understand what was required of him in the elicitation procedure, so most of the sessions were spent teaching him to read and spell. Very little progress was made with this as with his speech. However, he was clearly very pleased to be able to attend once a week as it allowed him to feel that someone was trying to do something for him. When he changed his job it was not possible for him to continue with his appointments. He had by then made forty visits. He completed the EPI with the questions being read out to him and his scores were 11 on neuroticism and 12 on extraversion.

I. FRANCIS

This thirty-nine year old man was referred through the psychiatric department of St. George's Hospital, where he was attending as an outpatient for treatment of a bout of depression. These depressive episodes were recurrent and were mainly characterized by early waking and a feeling of extreme exhaustion. He was taken on for treatment in spite of this psychiatric history because it was felt that the bouts of depression were not severe and appeared to be controlled by drugs.

He ran a family business selling children's clothing. Two of his sisters stuttered when they were young but were now fluent, and a paternal uncle still stutters. Previous treatment included a two-year attendance at group psychotherapy, which had not, he felt, greatly changed his stutter but he remarked that he had "learned a great deal about stuttering". In the middle of his treatment period he visited South Africa for six weeks during which time his stutter got considerably worse. On the Andrews-Harris Scale of Severity he was rated as Grade 2 (Moderate) at the start of treatment and Grade 1 (Mild) at the end, after attending for thirty-one sessions.

His speech was characterized by interjections, which he used before any word he anticipated having trouble with, and syllable repetitions. His scores on the EPI were 12 on neuroticism and 10 on extraversion and on the AH4 he had a verbal score of 40 and a performance score of 33 giving a total score of 73. Not only did this man's speech improve quite considerably but there was a marked change in his whole outlook on life, as perhaps can best be seen from the following extracts from his first and last self characterizations:

(a) (at the start of treatment)

> . . . He worries constantly of the impression he gives other people and tries to please and be popular in all forms of social intercourse . . . His stammer has prevented him from allowing his personality to develop to the full as a non-stammerer would be able to, and he feels unequal in an equal world.

(b) (at the end of treatment)

> . . . is today a confident, self sufficient person who through his strong determination plus sympathetic external help has become a useful member of society. He is now perfectly capable of taking his place in this tough competitive world. He is now leading a busy, active life and his life-long stammer that has dogged him has been largely overcome.
>
> People who meet him for the first time would find him mildly aggressive, but always prepared to be interested in other's problems. Lastly, he will not suffer fools gladly.

Follow-up

Periodic correspondence indicates that the reduction of 71% in total disfluencies and 68% in disfluent words has not only been maintained but improved upon up to three years since cessation of treatment.

J. REGINALD

This thirty-three year old man attended twenty-four times up until he and his family moved house, and it became too difficult for him to travel to London. His occupation was that of a garage mechanic. His family had told him that his stutter started at the age of eight years old, but gave him no specific cause and he was aware of no family history. He was married, had two children and was right-handed.

Once again there was a story of many attempts at treatment, including (a) group therapy for one year, (b) relaxation treatment for two to three months, (c) visits to a hypnotist who wanted him to attend twice a week, but which he found too expensive, (d) visits to a man who "just wanted my money—he pressed the bones in the back to put the nervous system in its proper place", and (e) a visit to someone who had appeared on television and who wanted £100 before starting treatment.

At the start of treatment Reginald's speech defect was rated as Grade 3 (Severe) on the Andrews-Harris scale and was still rated as Severe when he ceased to attend.

His defect took the form of repeating the first sound of the majority of words, sometimes for several minutes. He felt that the reduction in total disfluencies that was achieved (33%) was a real improvement. However, although there was a little more fluency, quite clearly he still had a very severe stutter. On the EPI he scored 17 on neuroticism and 8 on extraversion. On the AH4 he had a verbal and performance score of 30 giving a total score of 60. The following are two examples from his self characterizations:

(a) (at the start of treatment)

> ... is a man of quiet nature—that is, when he is with strangers and some of his friends, but when he is with his family and close friends he is the one who makes the conversation ... He does not mix very easily, because he is so self-conscious of his stammer. He relies on his wife too much, to do the talking when they are out shopping. He is always dreaming and hoping for things he knows are not likely ever to come his way.
>
> He is very happily married and has two lovely little girls—enough you would think to make anyone forget his worries—but not him; his stammer over-rules all that.

(b) (at the end of treatment)

> ... is very self conscious, who always thinks that people are talking or laughing about him especially as he has a stammer. He is rather a jovial person but if he should suspect anyone talking about him he then turns nasty and becomes very moody.

Follow-up

A reply to a follow-up letter revealed that he was having psychiatric treatment for a "nervous breakdown". He attributed this breakdown to his having many worries about his family and his speech, and said that since he had started psychiatric treatment, his worries were decreasing and this, in turn, was resulting in an improvement in his speech.

K. RONALD

When this eighteen year old young man came for treatment he was unmarried and worked as an adding machine repairer. During the thirty-six sessions he attended, his stuttering changed from Grade 2 (Moderate) to Grade 1 (Mild) and he was discharged prior to emigrating to Australia. This change in grade represents a reduction of more than 90% in disfluencies.

He believed he started stuttering at the age of five and reported that his father had a "mild stutter". Two previous attempts at treatment had involved relaxation and group therapy but had produced no lasting results. He was right-handed. His stutter consisted mainly of blocks, which he sought to break by increasing the volume of his speech, giving the impression that he was shouting. When he saw that his speech was steadily improving he decided to take the plunge and emigrate to Australia. He had always wanted to do this but he felt that it would be very difficult to get a job as long as his speech defect was so obtrusive. He had a neuroticism score of 20 and an extraversion score of 11 on the EPI. On the AH4 his verbal score was 26 and his performance score 39 giving a total score of 65.

Excerpts from two self characterizations

(a) (at the start of treatment)

> . . . is very moody and irritable, but not all the time. Most of the time he would rather stand back and listen when in strange company, rather than lead the conversation. The reason for this is because he has not got any self-confidence, and is afraid of showing himself up with his stuttering. He thinks everybody looks down on him and thinks he is stupid. He's got the idea that everybody is running him down. He's in a rut with his job and cannot get a better one because he hasn't got any drive. He is starting night school in September but he won't complete the course, but he is trying to convince himself he will. All in all he isn't much out of the ordinary—in fact he is a bit below average if anything.

(b) (at the end of treatment)

> . . . seems an average type of bloke—fairly easy to get on with. He's very good at his job, but not perfect. He is quite a likeable sort of chap really, but sometimes finds it difficult to express himself properly—mind you I always get the point he's trying to put across. He has not exactly got a stutter but there is the odd occasion when he gets a bit tongue-tied; apart from that he's as good as the next man.

Follow-up

There has been none due to his emigration to Australia.

L. PETER

This twenty-two year old motor mechanic attended forty-five times, at which point he said he wished to stop coming and go to a friend of his sister for treatment. He believed that he started stuttering severely at the age of six. His stutter at first testing was indeed so severe that for spontaneous speech he was only able to say seven words in four minutes. During the intervals between words he made breathing sounds, together with the occasional interjection "er" and the repetition of "a". The effort he put into speaking is best described by a note made on one occasion which read: "Stutter appalling today—silence for many seconds—tears pour out of his eyes with the effort to get the word out". He was right-handed and said his mother's father stuttered and so did his own father, but that the latter was now much better.

At start of treatment he was rated as Severe, Grade 3 (in fact he stuttered on 100% of the words) and was rated Grade 2 (Moderate) by the end of the 45th session. At the time he terminated treatment he was able to say fifty words in three minutes. So, although statistically there was a reduction of 86·5% of disfluent words and 66·1% of total dis-fluencies, he remained grossly handicapped because of the length of the blocks. He is a good example of the importance of including a measure of speed of speaking to insure a clear picture of the stuttering pattern. It was felt that his premature departure was unfortunate as there had been a definite change in his speech, and there did seem the remote possibility of further improvement, although the prognosis was not considered good with a speech defect of that severity.

Other treatments that his young man had tried were (a) hypnosis with no good effect; (b) visits to a private speech therapist who used "speech training", which he terminated as he felt he was getting nowhere; (c) another private speech therapist, who terminated the treatment her-self; (d) elocution classes; (e) another speech therapist. He said he wanted to have "another go" because he had heard of others getting some help. On the EPI he scored 2 on neuroticism and 8 on extraversion. The AH4 gave him a score of 25 on the verbal and 31 on the performance scale giving a total score of 56.

Extract from one self characterization

... He is a withdrawn sort of person because of his stammer, or maybe his stammer is just a symptom of this. Thus he is introverted, and not very mind-ful of other people except when they especially interest him. The first impres-sions he usually makes on a stranger is that of a rather stupid, tongue-tied person, who laughs too easily.

He is a slow and lethargic type, and unselfconfident in any activities re-quiring quick thought, i.e. conversation. He has a passive temperament, making him liable to be squashed by adversities rather than rising to their challenge.

His interests are rather limited—limited by his lack of energy and enthusi-asm. Apart from this he is a nice clean-cut young man.

Follow-up

In reply to a follow-up letter three years later he reports that his speech is much the same as it was. He is now attending group classes and finds it useful "meeting people with the same problem as myself".

M. ARNOLD

This young man was a twenty-one year old university student. At the first interview it transpired he thought he was going to have hypnosis, and was very disconsolate when he realized he was not. He was so insistent about having hypnosis that this was arranged for him, with the understanding that he could return to St. George's if he wished. In due course he did return and thought that, if anything, his speech was slightly worse.

There was no family history, he was right-handed, and believed he started stuttering at about five years of age. His previous treatments included (a) speech therapy lessons at school, where he was made to concentrate on vowels and specific consonants; (b) relaxation and practice in reading and speaking, which brought about some improvement in the treatment situation, but no generalization outside. He was convinced that he could cure himself if he "just had the confidence".

His scores on the EPI were 13 for neuroticism and for extraversion. On the AH4 he had a verbal score of 47 and a performance score of 44 giving a total score of 91. His speech was rated Grade 3 (Severe) on the Andrews-Harris scale both at the start and end of treatment. His speech defect was so severe that, in fact, the total disfluencies were unscorable. His syllable or part-word repetitions would go on for minutes during which time he would break off to take breath and then start again. Where Peter would have long periods of silence, this man filled the silences with a staccato sound. At the first testing he was able to say forty-five words in three minutes. He attended thirty-nine times until it was suggested to him that he was making no apparent progress and that perhaps he would be better going to someone else for treatment. It was arranged for a speech therapist to see him but he failed to keep any appointments.

On the Impgrid he was the only person to have a significant *negative* relationship between *like me in character* and *stutterers*—he was definitely not like other stutterers. This was perhaps reflected in his apparent unconcern about his very severe problem of communication.

Extract from a self characterization

> . . . is quite an easy person to become friendly with—he seems always eager to make friends, having once been approached—meaning that he seems very reserved and independent and yet when he is spoken to by someone in a friendly way he is very talkative in spite of his stammer—just in order to appear interesting and likeable.
>
> Once he has made friends with the person, this first intention of creating a good impression by being talkative and so slightly overcoming his stammer, gradually wears off. He has become used to the person and he usually finds them

uninteresting, boring or immature and so does not cherish the friendship. He then stammers much more—no longer intent on creating an impression, and perhaps seeking a new friendship.

He is a person who is never really satisfied with his "lot". He always wishes for things he is never likely to get or has no idea how to get it.

He has, I think, a slight sadistic characteristic. He judges somebody by looks, and out of about every dozen people (all men) he sees in a morning, he detests about four of them and feels like being rude to them or hitting them. I don't know why he feels like this—on the surface he seems a gentle sort of person . . .

N. ERIC

This man was a twenty-eight year old journalist, who was single and a migraine sufferer. He reported no family history of stuttering and was right-handed. The only previous attempt to eliminate his stutter consisted of speech therapy at the age of about eight which continued for some time.

His speech defect was characterized by an extraordinary ability to "avoid" stuttering. In ordinary conversation his stutter was virtually non-existent. He was above average in verbal fluency, and his speaking rate was above average. He only had a problem because his job entailed telephoning sports results to his newspaper, and as these inevitably involved the use of people's names, which he was unable to avoid, he stammered badly. The aims of treatment were therefore to persuade him to stop "avoiding" so that his view of himself as a stutterer could be discussed. While he was using avoidance techniques it was felt impossible to bring about any change. It was argued that he had predictions about stuttering which he never put to the test, and that it was only by doing so that modification of his 'stuttering' subsystem could be brought about. He could not do the S-grid as he appeared quite unable to think of himself stuttering in the presence of others.

He attended for twenty-nine sessions during which time his speaking rate was reduced from 135·6 to 112·2 words per minute, and he was able to read with no errors at all. His scores on the EPI were 7 on neuroticism and 12 on extraversion. On the AH4 his verbal score was 56 and his performance 52 giving a total score of 108.

O. RICHARD

This was a twenty-eight year old married man who was promoted from motor mechanic to foreman during the eighteen months in which he attended forty-five times. He attributed promotion to the improvement he was experiencing in his speech at that time which enabled him "to be himself".

His first attempt at treatment was at the age of eleven when he had attended group sessions for "speech correction". At the age of twenty-three he had group therapy again and then three years later had nine months of hypnosis. The only benefit he thought he had derived was from the hypnosis which helped reduce his anxiety. He thought he had stuttered all his speaking life and the only family history was of a cousin who stuttered.

The severity of his speech was rated as Grade 2 (Moderate) both at the start and end of treatment. However, the number of disfluent words *increased* during this period by 22·1%. The main characteristics of his speech were blocks and word repetitions. The severity of his stuttering fluctuated a great deal but appeared to improve overall quite considerably. However, talking into a tape recorder quite unnerved him and his stutter was far worse than at any other time. He was the only stutterer who, it was felt, had the severity of his speech substantially misrepresented by the recordings. His scores on the EPI were 4 for neuroticism and 16 for extraversion and on the AH4 he had a verbal score of 36 and a performance of 45 giving a total score of 81. He ceased to attend when a change of job took him away from London.

Follow-up

He failed to reply to all follow-up letters.

P. BRIAN

This young man was eighteen and had just left school. He was undecided whether to go to Technical College to get some Advanced level subjects or whether to do as his parents wished and go out to work. He had a maternal uncle who stuttered but no other family history and he was right-handed. His speech was characterized by blocks, which gave the unfortunate impression that he was being insolent and refusing to reply.

During the seventeen sessions he attended, his blocks became less obtrusive generally, and he said he found the effort of speaking was much less. On the Andrews-Harris scale the severity of his speech was rated Grade 1 (Mild) at the start and end of treatment, but within this category there was a reduction of 76% in disfluent words and 50% in total disfluencies. However, he had to travel a considerable distance each week to attend the hospital and it was decided that he should not attend for three months to see whether this improvement would continue without further help. He failed to answer any letters suggesting another appointment after the three months were up.

His scores on the EPI were 7 on neuroticism and 10 on extraversion. On the AH4 he had a verbal score of 42 and a performance score of 41 giving a total score of 83.

Q. CHRISTOPHER

This man was single, twenty-four years of age and a self-employed decorator. There was no family history of stuttering and he was right-handed. He had had one attempt at speech therapy but had received no benefit and subsequently tried to cure himself by reading books on the subject.

His main complaint was "difficulty in explaining things" and the fact that the words would come out too fast for him to pronounce them properly so that he stumbled over them. He was subsequently diagnosed by a speech therapist as a clutterer rather than a stutterer. According to Rieber and Froeschels (1966) the term was first used by Sheridan in 1762. Langova and Moravek (1964) reported finding abnormal electroencephalographic findings in 50% of a group of clutterers and atypical ones in 11%. Seeman (1966) is of the opinion that inter- and intra-verbal acceleration are the most typical symptoms of cluttering. Van Dantzig (1939) likened cluttering to typewriting when typing cannot keep pace with thought processes typical typing errors occur.

Christopher's speed of speaking was reduced by ten words per minute during the twenty-one sessions he attended but from then on he failed to keep any appointments. Subsequent correspondence revealed that he would have liked some guarantee that he would benefit from the treatment. He had to travel some distance, necessitating his losing half a day's work and, as he was self-employed, this was an important factor. Since no guarantee of improvement could be given, he did not attend again.

His scores on the EPI were 16 on neuroticism and 8 on extraversion he had a verbal score of 14 and a performance score of 26 giving a total score of 40 on the AH4.

R. HILDA

This twenty-five year old woman was a part-time teacher, unmarried, who lived with her mother. There was no family history and she was right-handed. She believed her stutter started at about the age of four or five. The only previous treatment she had had was from a speech therapist at school and, as far as she could remember, there was no demonstrable improvement.

Her speech was characterized by syllable repetitions and, on the Andrews-Harris scale, was rated Grade 2 (Moderate) at the start and end of treatment with considerable fluctuation throughout the time she attended. She gave up attending after thirty-nine sessions because her new-found business interests meant she had not sufficient time and also because there seemed to be no consistent improvement. The only thing to change substantially was her attitude. She became generally happier about her speech commenting "if I stammer that's just too bad". Her scores on the EPI were 9 on neuroticism and 12 on extraversion and on the AH4 she had a verbal score of 42 and a performance score of 51 giving a total score of 93. Overall change in disfluencies was minimal, only 3% in disfluent words and 5% in total disfluencies.

She experienced very great difficulty in doing the implications grids and also the self characterizations. For the latter she resorted to giving several descriptions of herself as seen through the eyes of various friends because she did not "know" who she was. Hilda was not well suited to this approach because of a general reluctance to talk about herself in anything but superficial terms. Early on in treatment, when the total inability to get a word out would force her to resort to writing down what she wanted to say, she would tear up the pieces of paper at the end of each session and put them in her handbag: "they are nobody's business but mine".

Follow-up

Three years later she rates herself as 'slightly better' than she was.

S. GORDON

At fifty years of age, this man was the oldest in the sample. He was a successful business man, married, who had stuttered since he began to speak. He had been given speech exercises about twelve years previously and had later had six sessions of hypnosis but derived little benefit from these approaches. His maternal grandmother stuttered and so did his thirteen year old son. It was arranged for his son to receive treatment from a speech therapist and he responded well.

Gordon's speech defect changed steadily from being Severe (Grade 3) to Moderate (Grade 2) during the sixty-one occasions on which he attended. This change in grade represented a reduction of 68% in disfluent words and 67% in total disfluencies. The outstanding features of his speech defect were very long-sustained prolongations and all forms of repetition.

His scores on the EPI were 15 on neuroticism and 5 on extraversion. On the AH4 he had a verbal score of 38 and a performance score of 42 giving a total score of 80.

Extract from one self characterization

... rather inclined to self pity and to find an easy excuse in blaming a speech impediment for not being as successful as he would wish. He would presumably be more successful in his job if he did not worry about his stammer so much and developed more outside interests ... Can be a good friend and understanding companion, but inclined to become moody and "dry up" if he feels his stammer is particularly bad ...

Follow-up

At a nine-months follow-up he had maintained the improvement but still reported getting "stuck" on certain words, although now he said he rarely worried about them. He remarked that one of the big changes which he was very pleased about was that he no longer "got tied up" when speaking with his son.

He failed to reply to a letter at the three-year follow-up.

T. LUKE

Luke's sessions were tape-recorded throughout and these have been used as the basis for presenting the therapeutic process described in Chapter 9.

III. COMMENT

As individuals, these people were as different from or as similar to, any other group of twenty people. But they can be compared to others on the basis of measures used. For instance, they were well above average in intelligence *as a group*, although several individuals were well below average. *As a group* they were not substantially more introverted or neurotic than the general population. One other point worth commenting on is that *as a group* their speech disorder was much more severe than that reported in other samples. For instance, the mean number of total disfluencies (42·06) at the first testing approach the 9th percentile in Johnson's (Johnson *et. al.*, 1963) data (44·9). There is a definite impression that this type of approach to stuttering is very much less successful if the stutter is severe—there is less fluency for the stutterer to experiment with. If this is so, then better results would have been achieved with a more "average" group. However, this was an unselected group and the results must be assessed accordingly.

CHAPTER 7

The Results

Many people used to believe that angels moved the stars. It now appears that they do not. As a result of this and like revelations, many people do not now believe in angels.

R. D. Laing (1967)

I. ANALYSIS OF IMPLICATIONS GRIDS

A. SCORING OF IMPLICATIONS

Implications Counts

It was possible that the total number of implications in a grid might be a simple function of the number of constructs elicited. To check on this, correlations were run between the *absolute* number of implications used by an individual and the *average* number for each construct. The Spearman rho correlations between these two methods of scoring were 0·85 and 0·91 for the S- and NS-grids respectively. Since these two scores had such a substantial proportion of their variance in common, *absolute* number of implications has been used in all statistical comparisons, unless otherwise stated.

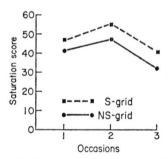

FIG. 9.   Group mean "saturation" scores for S- and NS-grids on three test occasions.

Implications Saturation

The term "saturation" refers to the degree to which the number of implications obtained on a specific grid is related to the total number possible in a grid of that size. That is to say, for a grid with ten bi-polar

114

constructs, the total number of implications possible would be one hundred and eighty (10×20 minus the diagonals). If an individual "saw" ninety interconstruct implications, he would have a saturation score of 50%.

Figure 9 shows how little difference in saturation there was, for the group as a whole, between the two types of grid and between test occasions. However, certain differences do appear when intra-group differences are examined and these are discussed later.

B. S- AND NS-IMPGRID COMPARISONS

Differences in Numbers of Implications

Changes in mean number of implications for "stutterer" (S) and "nonstutterer" (NS) grids can be seen in Fig. 10. On the first test occasion the

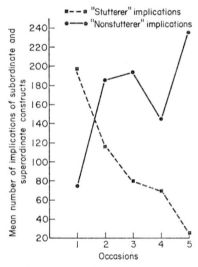

Fig. 10. Group mean number of implications for subordinate and superordinate constructs on S- and NS-grids on five test occasions. Occasions 1–5: N=18, 16, 8, 4, 2 respectively (solid line); N=19, 15, 6, 3, 2 respectively (dashed line).

difference between the total number of implications for the two types of grid was significant at the 1% level. At the start of treatment the stutterers were better able to construe themselves as *stutterers* than as nonstutterers. If one takes the total number of implications as an operational definition of *meaningfulness*, then being a stutterer was significantly more meaningful. Because of the small number of stutterers completing more than three grids, the data from grids 3, 4, and 5 are pooled. A comparison of these pooled data between the S- and NS-grids shows again that they differ significantly ($p < 0.05$*) in their number of implications or meaningfulness. This suggests that towards the end of treatment the members of the group as a whole were better able to construe themselves as *nonstutterers* than as stutterers, representing a highly significant reversal from their construing at the start of treatment.

The total number of NS implications rose significantly from first to last testing ($p < 0.005$) but the decrease in S implications did not reach significance due to the very large individual variation.

Superordinacy

A superordinate construct has been operationally defined as a construct which has been "laddered" from another. Although this operational definition has some experimental support (Hinkle, 1965), it does not always match well with other theoretically-derived operational definitions of superordinacy (Bannister and Salmon, 1967). However, bearing in mind the problems of interpretation, Hinkle's method for defining superordinacy was used as a basis for comparison of the mean number of implications for superordinate and subordinate constructs ($a + b$ and $c + d$ in Fig. 11) on S- and NS-grids.

a Subordinate Implications of SUBORDINATE Constructs	b Superordinate Implications of SUBORDINATE Constructs
c Subordinate Implications of SUPERORDINATE Constructs	d Superordinate Implications of SUPERORDINATE Constructs

FIG. 11. Schematic representation of construct and implication superordinacy for the implications grids.

On Occasion I, not only do the S-grids contain more than twice the number of all types of implication at first testing, but they also have a higher *ratio* of implications for superordinate constructs than for subordinate constructs. If one argues that superordinate constructs give a

* No predictions were made concerning the S-grids, so two-tail tests of significance were used on the T values from the Wilcoxon Matched-Paired Signed-Ranks Test.

person a certain degree of freedom from the detailed events of life, then one can interpret the data in Fig. 12 as indicating that the stutterer has a more workable and flexible as well as a more extensive sub-system to do with himself as a stutterer than as a fluent speaker at the start of treatment.

The development of the rudimentary NS system would be expected also to result in an increase of superordinate over subordinate implications, if it is to become equally as workable and as flexible as the previously dominating S system. The data shown in Fig. 12 suggest that this

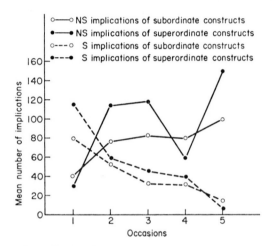

FIG. 12.   Mean numbers of subordinate and superordinate construct implications on S- and NS-grids on five test occasions.

may, indeed, be the case. The drop on Occasion 4 in NS implications for superordinate constructs cannot be accounted for except in terms of individual variation. Only four stutterers completed grids at this stage of treatment and two of these were showing marked fluctuation at the time.

Inter- and Intra-Construct Correlations

The significant correlations between numbers of implications on the two types of grid on the first occasion and change from first to last occasion, can be seen in Table II. Since the number of people completing the grids decreased with time, the level at which the correlations are significant varies. Unless otherwise stated, the correlations given are significant at the 5% level.

There is a tendency for the absolute number of implications given by each person to be related on the S- and NS-grids ($r_s = 0.44$); if a high number is given on one grid, there is a likelihood of there being a high number on the other. As there was this individual consistent tendency, a percentage measure of change was used as well as the absolute score. Thus, a person starting out with 100 implications and increasing these to 120 would have the same absolute increase as another starting out with 20 and increasing to 40, but the first person would have an increase of 20% and the other of 100%.

TABLE II

Significant correlations (r_s) between numbers of S and NS implications on (a) the first test occasion and (b) change from first to last testing.

	1	2	3	4	5	6
1. NS 1	—	—	—	0·44	—	—
2. NS last minus first			0·81 + +		−0·77 + +	−0·74
3. NS last minus first %				—	−0·45	−0·51
4. S1					0·56	—
5. S last minus first					—	0·93 + +
6. S last minus first %						

+ + $p < 0.01$

However, the correlations between *absolute* and *percentage* measures of change for both S- and NS-grids show there to be considerable similarity between these two methods of scoring ($r_s = 0.93$ and 0.81 respectively). But the need for discriminating between them is shown by the fact that the significant correlation of 0·56 between initial *absolute* number of S implications and reduction in number from first to last testing, is not reflected in the *percentage* measure. A person starting out with a large number of implications has more room for manoeuvre, he has more to decrease. No significant relationship exists between amount of change and initial number of NS implications.

Both *absolute* and *percentage* measures also show a tendency for the change in number of implications to vary similarly in both S- and NS-grids—the more a stutterer changed on one type of grid, the more inclined he was to change on the other, but in the opposite direction.

Summary

1. The number of implications to do with being a nonstutterer increased during the course of treatment.
2. There were significantly *fewer* nonstutterer implications than stutterer implications at the start of treatment.
3. There were significantly *more* nonstutterer than stutterer implications at the end of treatment.

4. The increase in nonstutterer implications during the treatment period was significant but the decrease in stutterer implications was not, due to wide individual variation.
5. At the start of treatment, S-grids had a higher ratio of superordinate to subordinate implications than the NS-grids.
6. The *absolute* numbers of implications on the two types of grid were related—there was an individual tendency to give many or few.
7. The degree of change in number of implications was related on both grids.
8. There was no difference in saturation scores (total number of implications given in relation to total number possible) between the two types of grid and between test occasions *for the group as a whole.*

C. IMPLICATIONS AND INTELLIGENCE

One of the most consistent findings from research using the rank order form of repertory grid technique is the lack of a significant relationship between intelligence and grid measures. However, there is no information as yet concerning any possible relationship between intelligence and scores derived from implications grids. Correlations were therefore calculated between initial number of S and NS implications and intelligence (full score on the AH4). For initial number of S implications, the correlation with intelligence was 0·09, but that for NS implications was −0·65 ($p < 0.01$). All sorts of arguments could be put forward to account for this rather unexpected finding. For instance, a correlation of this size is going to occur every one hundred times by chance alone, and this could be one such time. Or else, it could be the result of an artefact (unspecified) of the conditions in which the constructs and implications were elicited.

Assuming that it is not an artefact nor a chance occurrence, one can speculate further. With the S-grid, the stutterer is being asked to give constructs he uses in his relationships with others. But in deriving the NS constructs he is being asked to speculate. The more severe his stutter, the more speculative will be his construing. He has to imagine himself as a nonstutterer talking to people who are like him in that they are also fluent. This correlation suggests that the more intelligent the person, the less able (or willing) he is to speculate in this fashion. This group of stutterers consisted, on the whole, of people of above average intelligence when compared with the population in general (see Table I, p. 95).

This unwillingness to speculate about a more or less hypothetical situation had no direct effect on the stutterer's ability to change his construing over time (r_s IQ versus per cent change in NS implications = −0·09), nor in his response to treatment (r_s IQ versus per cent change in disfluent words = −0·38), although the direction of the relationships is negative. One is left with the simple statement that, for this group of stutterers, the more intelligent the person, the fewer implications he was likely to see between the constructs he used for construing himself as a nonstutterer.

D. CONSTRUCT CONTENT ANALYSIS

In all, forty-five "stutterer" and forty-eight "nonstutterer" grids were completed, the former containing two hundred and ten constructs and the latter two hundred and forty-five constructs.

One of the major problems facing anyone wanting to categorize elicited constructs is that verbal labels are not necessarily the same as constructs. The difference between two constructs with the same verbal labels often becomes clearly apparent when their implications and their opposites are considered. In 1965, Landfield produced a manual providing a basis on which constructs could be divided into twenty-two categories (forty-two sub-categories) giving definitions and descriptive examples. He later reported (Landfield, 1967) the interjudge reliability of some of these categories and indicated those in which there was either 75% or 65% agreement among judges as to the appropriate category for a particular construct.

An attempt was made in this study to categorize the elicited constructs given by the stutterers under Landfield's twenty-two headings. It was considered necessary for an independent rater to carry out this task as the author was too familiar with the stutterers and their construing to be sure of being wholly objective. This classification of constructs is purely for descriptive purposes. It is of some interest to establish, as accurately as possible, the types of constructs a fairly heterogeneous group of English stutterers apply to themselves and others, and to compare these with any other normative data as they become available.

The independent rater was given the manual and simply told to go ahead and categorize the constructs according to the instructions. This proved to be a far more difficult task than had at first appeared. While the majority of constructs gave no real problem, the rater considered that a substantial minority could be put in any one of several categories. It was decided that the appropriate category for a construct with an ambiguous emergent pole should be determined by its implicit pole (i.e. its opposite). No attempt was made to assess the reliability of the groupings so obtained.

Analysis I

Details of the categorization of these constructs for the group as a whole are given in Appendix 2. Level of interjudge reliability (as quoted by Landfield) is given with each construct category. With each sub-category is detailed (i) the number of stutterers from whom the construct was elicited; (ii) the number of constructs which were superordinate or subordinate; (iii) where possible, whether the responses came mainly from S- or NS-grids; if the construct occurred in both types of grid, this is indicated by "both"; in some cases the opposite pole of a construct is given where it is regarded as rather atypical.

The emergent pole is stated in all cases. For instance, thirteen stutterers did not all use the single word "sympathetic" as the emergent pole in the Tenderness category, but the words used appeared sufficiently

TABLE III

Relationships for one stutterer between the constructs *stutterer–nonstutterer* and *self–not self* and the emergent poles of three constructs on S- and NS-grids on five test occasions. (+ = positive, − = negative, 0 = construct not elicited.)

	Stutterer	Non-stutterer	Self	Not Self	Stutterer	Non-stutterer	Self	Not Self
		SHY/RESERVED				MIX WELL		
S1	0	−	+	−	0	0	0	0
S2	0	0	0	0	0	0	0	0
S3	+	0	0	−	−	0	−	+
S4	0	0	0	0	0	0	0	0
S5	0	0	0	0	0	0	0	0
NS1	+	0	+	−	0	0	+	−
NS2	0	0	0	0	0	0	−	+
NS3	0	0	0	0	0	0	+	−
NS4	+	0	+	−	0	0	+	−
NS5	0	0	0	0	0	0	0	0
		WEAK						
S1	0	0	0	0				
S2	+	0	0	0				
S3	0	0	0	0				
S4	+	0	0	0				
S5	+	0	0	0				
NS1	0	0	0	0				
NS2	0	0	0	0				
NS3	+	−	0	0				
NS4	+	0	−	−				
NS5	+	0	0	0				

alike to the rater to be grouped under the single verbal label. When a construct appeared in several grids of the same person, it was counted only once. Certain information is lost as the result of this procedure since changes in the construing of *self* and *stutterer* are expected to occur as the role of fluent speaker becomes more familiar. Table III gives an indication of the degree of variation that was found across grids of the same person in the presence or absence of three poles of different constructs.

The categories of External Appearance and Factual Description have few entries because, during elicitation, the stutterers were encouraged to produce more "psychological" constructs. This was done by agreeing that, for instance, *dark-haired–light-haired* was one important way in which two of the people differed from the third, but then asking if there were not some other important basis for making a discrimination.

Analysis 2

All the constructs elicited from each individual were then categorized and the number falling into each category stated as a percentage of the total for that person. The figures in Table IV are the mean percentage of total constructs falling in each category for the present sample of nineteen stutterers as compared with the mean percentage for thirty American college students reported in Landfield (1971).

Landfield's figures are the mean percentages of fifteen constructs given for any one category by twelve male and eighteen female American college students. The present comparison is an imperfect one since Landfield omitted five categories which gave unsatisfactory interjudge consistency correlations. However, since only 6·4% of the stutterers' responses fell into these categories, the effect would be to enhance the following three very obvious differences between the two samples. First, the American sample has considerably more *active* (e.g. talkative, extrovert) than inactive (e.g. withdrawn, shy) Social Interaction constructs. For the stutterers this is reversed. More than one quarter of all their responses relate to *inactive* social interactions. Second, the stutterers give twice as many High Status constructs (e.g. ambitious, educated) and, thirdly, twice as many High Intellective constructs (e.g. intelligent, wise) than the American students.

The most likely interpretation of the high proportion of constructs to do with social interaction among the stutterer group is that the triadic elicitation procedure was specifically designed to encourage the construing of the self in social interaction with others. That 39·2% of all responses fell in the Social Interaction category is taken as an indication that the aim of the elicitation procedure was at least partially fulfilled. The fact that the majority of emergent construct poles described socially

TABLE IV

Comparison of the mean percentage of constructs occurring in each category (Landfield, 1965) for 19 stutterers and 30 American college students.

Category			LANDFIELD SAMPLE Mean % total responses (N = 30)	FRANSELLA SAMPLE Mean % total responses (*N* = 19)	
Social interaction	high	1a	11	11·6⎫	social
	low	1b	1	27·6⎭	interaction
Forcefulness	high	2a	14	10·8	
	low	2b	6	3·8	
Organization	high	3a	3	1·7	
	low	3b	3	1·0	
Self-sufficiency	high	4a	2	1·8	
	low	4b	3	1·6	
Status	high	5a	3	6·0⎫	status
	low	5b	2	2·4⎭	
Factual description		6	1	0·7	
Intellective	high	7a	3	6·1⎫	intellective
	low	7b	2	1·7⎭	
Self reference		8	0	0·0	
Imagination	high	9a	—	0·3	
	low	9b	1	0·2	
Alternatives– alternatives		10a	—	0·6	
inferable alternatives		10b	5	0·3	
Sexual		11	0	0·8	
Morality	high	12a	3	3·1	
	low	12b	3	0·7	
External appearance		13	1	0·7	
Emotional arousal		14	7	7·3	
Diffuse generalization		15	—	2·6	
Egoism	high	16a	3	3·0	
	low	16b	—	1·6	
Tenderness	high	17a	4	3·6	
	low	17b	5	1·0	low tenderness
Time orientation	past	18a	0	1·0	
	future	18b	1	0·8	
	present	18c	—	0·9	
Involvement	high	19a	3	2·5	
	low	19b	3	2·0	
Comparatives		20	—	0·4	
Extreme qualifiers		21	3	0·0	
Humour	high	22a	1	1·2	
	low	22b	1	0·2	

inactive interaction can be understood, on common sense grounds, as likely to occur among those who have problems of communication. Stutterers focus on, and fret about, not being able to interact with others as they would wish. The emphasis on status and intellectual powers perhaps reflects the stutterer's concern about his role relationships and his tendency to think people regard him as a rather dull, mediocre person (that is when he is being "the stutterer").

Analysis 3

Stutterers do not always construe themselves *as stutterers* along the same dimensions as they construe themselves *as people* (Fransella, 1968). They agree that, when speaking, they share certain characteristics with other stutterers but otherwise they are not like "them". An attempt has been made to look at this further by analysing all the constructs that were used by ten or more of the group. If there were no differences between the construing of *self as a person* and *self as a stutterer*, then it would be expected that if, say, *like me in character* implied being *impulsive*, then being *a stutterer* should also imply being *impulsive*. Similarly, if being *not like me in character* implied being *not impulsive* then being *a non-stutterer* might also be expected to imply being *not impulsive*.

As a rough measure of the degree to which there was concordance between *stutterer* and *self* constructs and *nonstutterer* and *not self* constructs, frequency tables for the various combinations of response were compiled and are given in Appendix 3. Since the person was not compelled to say there definitely *was* an implied relationship between any two constructs, the number of nil responses is also given.

Two things emerge fairly clearly from this analysis. First, there is surprisingly little agreement between the construct dimensions used for construing the *self* and those used for construing *stutterers*. Second, the "nil" response category is used far more often than any other category and applies more often to the construct *stutterer* than to *self*. Since the analysis is of constructs used by more than half the sample, it is perhaps surprising that they are not applied more often in *self* and *stutterer* construing.

Further evidence that stutterers do not see themselves as such is to be found in the fact that only five out of nineteen in the group had a significant positive relationship on *any* of their grids between *like me in character* and *stutterers*. Arnold, the most severe stutterer, had a significant *negative* relationship between the two constructs—he was definitely *not* like other stutterers. Out of the six stutterers who definitely either did or did not see themselves as they see other stutterers, five failed to reduce their disfluencies by as much as 50% *or* terminated treatment prematurely. The sixth showed the greatest amount of improvement. There thus seems a suggestion that construing the self along the *stutterer* dimension contra-indicates substantial improvement, although the fact that one who did identify himself as a stutterer showed the greatest amount of improvement must be borne in mind.

It is perhaps worth noting that all these attempts at analysing constructs must be of descriptive value only. Landfield has made a start at what is a very complex matter and a great deal more work will need to be done before anything meaningful can be said with confidence about differences between groups in the types of constructs they use and, more particularly, how they use them.

Summary

1. For descriptive purposes only, the four hundred and fifty-five constructs used on the ninety-three Impgrids by nineteen stutterers were categorized using Landfield's method of analysis.
2. The constructs were categorized for each individual and the mean percentages of constructs falling in each of Landfield's categories were compared with his normative data. The stutterer group gave large numbers of Socially Inactive Interaction constructs, and about twice as many High Status and High Intellective constructs as a group of American college students.
3. Stutterers do not necessarily construe themselves and stutterers as a group along the same construct dimensions—they do not see themselves as stutterers.

II. ANALYSIS OF SPEECH DISFLUENCIES

Three measures were taken from tape recorded speech samples. Each stutterer, at intervals throughout his treatment, recorded reading from a standard passage of prose and three minutes, spontaneous speech. Two measures were of disfluencies and the third of rate of utterance, i.e. the number of words spoken in one minute.

A. RATE OF UTTERANCE

The number of stutterers in each comparison of rate of speaking or reading is eighteen and not twenty. For both Eric, the "avoider" and Susan, the rapid speaker, the aim was to decrease rather than increase the rate of speaking. The same applied to Eric for reading (but not Susan who stuttered badly while reading) and Andrew, who was illiterate and had to be left out of the calculations.

The means and standard deviations for reading and speaking rates on the first and last test occasions are shown in Table V. The correlation between speaking and reading rates on the first test occasion was 0·74 and is somewhat lower than that of 0·90 reported by Sander (1961) but is still highly significant.

TABLE V

Means and Standard Deviations for three measures of speaking and reading: time in words per minute, total disfluencies per 100 words, disfluent words per 100 words.

| | | Speaking | | Reading | |
		Mean	S.D.	Mean	S.D.
Time in w.p.m.	First	82·40	50·76	55·30	39·74
	Last	90·07	50·75	69·53	42·02
Total disfluencies	First	42·06	52·23	37·88	39·09
per 100 words	Last	16·93	24·96	20·02	23·89
Disfluent words	First	18·55	28·73	18·75	21·15
per 100 words	Last	10·33	21·94	11·89	13·72

Change in Rate of Utterance Over the Treatment Period

The correlation of 0·74 between reading and speaking rate on the first test occasion drops to 0·47 when change in rate of reading and speaking from first to last testing is compared. This indicates that all the stutterers did not increase their rate of utterance to the same extent on both speaking tasks.

Neither initial rate of reading or speaking was predictive of the amount of change likely to occur ($-0·22$ and $-0·34$ respectively). But the amount of increase in rate of speaking from before to after treatment is highly significant ($p < 0·005$)* and just significant for reading ($p < 0·05$).*

Comparison with Normative Data

The relative severity of speech disorder for the group as a whole can be assessed by comparing the mean rate of speaking with some normative data provided by Johnson *et al.*, (1963). The mean rate for the present group changed from being just above the 3rd decile rank at the start of treatment to just below the 4th decile rank at the end of treatment when compared with Johnson's stutterers—they were a group with very slow rate of speaking at the start and were still comparatively slow at the finish. Whether such cross-cultural comparisons are valid is not known. It may well be that Americans are faster speakers than Britons and that

---

* Wilcoxon Matched-Pairs Signed-Ranks Test; one-tail test of significance.

their stutterers speak more quickly. But the present group were also found to have more disfluencies than the average American stutterer, which is consistent with the finding concerning their general slowness. The present data are also similar to those reported for the Newcastle upon Tyne sample (Andrews and Harris 1964) suggesting that there may be a cultural difference.

B. DISFLUENCY ANALYSIS

The means and standard deviations for disfluent words and total disfluencies are given in Table V and the intercorrelations in Table VI.

TABLE VI

Correlations between two measures of disfluency in reading and speaking at first testing (I) and for percentage change from first and last testing.

		2	3	4	5	6	7	8
Reading (I)— disfluent words	1	$0·67^{++}$	$0·86^{++}$	$0·70^{++}$	$-0·33$	$-0·12$	$-0·37$	$-0·30$
Speaking (I)— disfluent words	2		$0·79^{++}$	$0·92^{++}$	$-0·50$	$-0·14$	$-0·39$	$0·03$
Reading (I)— total disfluencies	3			$0·73^{++}$	$-0·45^{+}$	$-0·33$	$-0·32$	$-0·32$
Speaking (I)— total disfluencies	4				$-0·48^{+}$	$-0·14$	$-0·39$	$0·22$
Reading— disfluent words first–last %	5					$0·36$	$0·90^{++}$	$0·22$
Speaking— disfluent words first–last %	6						$0·40^{+}$	$0·59^{+}$
Reading— total disfluencies first–last %	7							$0·38$
Speaking— total disfluencies first–last % minus	8							

$^{+}$ $p < 0·05$
$^{++}$ $p < 0·01$

Disfluent words versus total disfluencies

Intercorrelations at first testing. At the first testing, disfluent words and total disfluencies correlated significantly both for speaking ($r_s = 0·92$) and for reading ($r_s = 0·86$). Sander's comparable correlations were 0·87 and 0·86. Those between initial reading and speaking were 0·67 for disfluent words and 0·73 for total disfluencies—again very similar to those reported by Sander (0·72 and 0·70 respectively).

Intercorrelations for Degree of Change. From first to last testing the *amount of change* on the two measures (disfluent words and total disfluencies) correlated 0·90 for reading but only 0·59 for speaking. While this latter correlation is statistically significant at the 1% level, the two measures have only 35% of their variance in common. One reason for this rather lower correlation between the two measures when assessing change in speaking disfluencies is to be found in the atypical behaviour of one person. Susan (the rapid speaker) totally eliminated her disfluent words but made few inroads on her interjections, revisions and other types of disfluency only counted in the total disfluency measure. Without her the correlation between the two measures of change in speaking disfluency would have been 0·71.

Sander (1961) comments on the great variability in his stutterers' fluency after only a twenty-four hour interval, and how reading and speaking errors do not fluctuate together. In the present sample, a similar lack of consistency is reflected in the correlations between change in reading and speaking disfluencies of 0·36 for disfluent words and 0·38 for total disfluencies.

Inspection of the scores of those yielding large differences in the ranked order of disfluent words and total disfluencies shows that they tended to maintain their initial number of interjections, word and phrase repetitions and revisions (all included in the total disfluency but not in the disfluent word score), while decreasing the other disfluencies. The low correlation for total disfluency change between reading and speaking could be accounted for by the fact that interjections, word and phrase repetitions and revisions are less likely to occur in reading. But this would not account for the low correlation for change in number of disfluent words between reading and speaking. It was certainly observed that, in some cases, speech generally became markedly more fluent during speaking than reading and sometimes reading had to be practiced as if it were a separate skill.

Disfluencies as Predictors of Change. In general, initial level of disfluency turned out to be a poor predictor of subsequent change. The only consistency in the correlations is that both measures of disfluencies in speaking and one in reading show that the higher the level of initial disfluency, the less likelihood there is of there being a reduction in disfluent words during reading. Nearly all correlations, in fact, show a negative relationship between initial level of severity and subsequent improvement, but only one reaches significance. This is partly the result of the two most severe stutterers leaving before the end of their treatment. But it is also probable that the severe stutterer is less likely to improve with this treatment approach since he has less fluency upon which to build.

Comparisons with Normative Data. Apart from assessing the degree of absolute change in disfluency scores, the means were compared with the ranges and decile ranks of distributions of total disfluencies per hundred words that are provided in Johnson *et al.*, (1963). The normative data for reading errors could not be used since the reading passages employed in the present study differed from Johnson's. For the group as a whole, the mean total disfluency score of 42·06 at first testing of spontaneous speech falls between the 7th percentile (29·6) and the 8th percentile (44·9) for Johnson's sample of fifty male stutterers. The range of disfluencies of the present sample is from 0·8 to 157·0 compared with Johnson's 2·7 to 127·3. The present group can therefore be considered to consist of more severe stutterers than the American sample in terms of total disfluencies. This is consistent with the finding that they are more severe also as measured by their speed of speaking.

Degree of Disfluency Change Over the Treatment Period. Table VII sets out the levels at which the different measures of speech show the group to have significantly reduced its number of disfluencies. The extent of the reduction on all measures can be assessed as well from the fact that at the last testing the mean total disfluency score of 16·9, falls between Johnson's 4th percentile (15·1) and the 5th (19·0), showing there to have been a fall of three decile ranks for the group as a whole.

TABLE VII

Results of the Wilcoxon Matched-Pairs Signed-Ranks Test applied to change on two measures of disfluency between initial and final testing.

		T	P
Disfluent words—speaking	(N = 19)	12	<0·005
Disfluent words—reading	(N = 18)	17	<0·005
Total disfluencies—speaking	(N = 18)	6	<0·005
Total disfluencies—reading	(N = 18)	28·5	<0·01

Taking a 50% reduction in speech errors on the speaking test as significant improvement, then 63% or ten out of sixteen stutterers improved on the total disfluency measure and 69% on the disfluent word count. If significant improvement is taken to be a decrease in disfluencies of more than 50% on *either* measure, then 81% or thirteen out of sixteen improved.

It may look like special pleading to take the number of stutterers in the group as only sixteen, but it is argued that to include the others would be to mistake rigidity for scientific purity. One stutterer was unscorable at the start and at the end of treatment. Maybe he did reduce his errors on the total disfluency measure by more than 50%, but there was no way of knowing. However, there are grounds for including him in with the disfluent word scorers in view of the fact that he could be said to have stuttered on one hundred words in one hundred on both test occasions. In this case, 63% and not 69% can be said to have significantly improved. As for the other three: Eric, the "avoider", was expected to increase and not decrease his disfluencies on both measures—which he did; Andrew could not be said to have undergone treatment since his illiteracy meant that each session was largely devoted to the teaching of reading; and Christopher was diagnosed as a clutterer and could therefore not be regarded as a member of the stutterer sample.

TABLE VIII

Change in disfluencies during treatment. (i) Change in decile ranks for speaking rate and total disfluencies based on data provided by Johnson *et al.*, (1963) and (ii) percent change in total disfluencies and disfluent words.

	Speaking rate decile rank			Speaking total disfluencies decile rank			Total disflu- encies	Dis- fluent words
	1st	last	change	1st	last	change	% change	% change
1. William	2	9	7	7	1	6	93·7	95·7
2. Luke	2	7	5	7	2	5	71·1	64·0
3. Mary	2	8	6	4	1	3	54·0	32·5
4. Geoffrey	3	7	4	4	1	3	87·2	100·0
5. John	2	2	0	6	3	3	43·4	80·0
6. Susan	9	9	0	1	1	0	25·3	100·0
7. Michael	6	8	2	5	1	4	70·0	38·0
8. Henry	7	4	−3	1	1	0	15·4	81·0
9. Andrew*	2	2	0	6	4	2	33·7	−11·2
10. Francis	4	7	3	5	1	4	71·1	68·0
11. Reginald	1	1	0	9	9	0	32·7	13·1
12. Ronald	2	5	3	9	1	8	96·2	91·7
13. Peter	1	1	0	9	8	1	66·1	86·5
14. Arnold	1	1	0	—	—	—	—	—
15. Eric**	8	6	−2	1	4	−3	−74·4	−84·6
16. Richard	1	1	0	8	8	0	−18·6	−22·1
17. Brian	3	6	3	1	1	0	50·4	75·9
18. Christopher***	8	7	−1	2	1	1	5·5	37·8
19. Hilda	6	7	1	3	3	0	5·4	3·0
20. Gordon	1	3	2	9	5	4	67·0	67·6

* Illiterate
** "Avoider"
*** Clutterer

Table VIII gives details of change for the individuals who received treatment. It can be seen that 56·3% changed their decile rank by three or more places and, of those who improved significantly, some changed only moderately while others approached fluency. If one sees the therapeutic procedure as an attempt to show someone how to adopt a new way of life, then it is not surprising that he only "approaches" fluency. When the going gets tough, there is often a partial relapse for a short time—the stutterer retreats to his much more familiar pattern of speaking until the threat has past.

Follow-up information has already been given for each person in Chapter 6. But, in summary, contact was lost with ten of the nineteen stutterers: three went abroad and six ceased their treatment prematurely for a variety of reasons. For only one of those who completed their course of treatment is there no reason for failure to give a follow-up report.

Of the nine for whom follow-up data are available (the interval ranging from nine months to three years) four have continued to improve (two "very much"), two report further slight improvement, two "no change" and one "worse". The stutterer who reported being worse had shown little improvement during treatment and had to cease attending because of a move further away from London, and he subsequently had to seek psychiatric help.

One Measure or More? On the whole, the two measures of disfluency correlated very highly together. The question thus arises of whether both were necessary. Williams and Kent (1958) found that it was part-word repetitions and sound prolongations that were more likely to be judged as "stutters" by listeners, while revisions were likely to be judged as normal disfluencies. Young (1961) supported this finding by reporting that ratings of stuttering severity correlated 0·83 with part-word repetitions and 0·76 with sound prolongations but only 0·18 with revisions. This being the case, the disfluent word count seems the more appropriate as a measure of change in stuttering, since the more comprehensive total disfluency measure will be taking into account what, to the listener, may be judged as normal disfluencies.

Two other points favour the disfluent word measure. A disfluency is only counted once when it occurs on the same word. With a severe stutterer this is a great advantage. In Arnold's case, for example, it was impossible to count the number of total disfluencies since his syllable repetitions were so numerous—continuing on occasion for several minutes with just the occasional pause for breath. To calculate such repetitions was not only almost impossible, it was pointless. It was far more meaningful to give him a disfluent word score of 100 words stuttered out of 100 words spoken. A final factor in favour of the disfluent word count is that, having fewer categories, it is quicker and easier to use.

However, reducing one's measures usually involves loss of information. Discrepancies in reductions of disfluencies on the two measures gives information as to the type of change in stuttering pattern. A person with a 70% reduction in total disfluencies and only 38% in disfluent words is probably having many fewer repetitions on a similar number of words. Alternatively, figures of 15% reduction in total disfluencies and 81% in disfluent words suggests that very many more words are spoken fluently, but those that are stuttered involve as many disfluent utterances—probably part-word repetitions.

C. INTERACTION BETWEEN DISFLUENCIES AND RATE OF UTTERANCE

Intercorrelations between reading and speaking rates of utterance and disfluencies are given in Table IX. Sander's (1961) comparable data for reading and speaking rates with total disfluencies are 0·86 and 0·81 respectively.

TABLE IX

Correlations (r_s) between rate of utterance and two disfluency measures for reading and speaking at initial testing.

	Reading I w.p.m.	Speaking I w.p.m.
Reading disfluent words	−0·40*	−0·60**
Reading total disfluencies	−0·57**	−0·65**
Speaking disfluent words	−0·67**	−0·89**
Speaking total disfluencies	−0·61**	−0·88**

* $p < 0·05$
** $p < 0·01$.

Both rate of reading and of speaking at the start of treatment were significantly predictive of per cent change in disfluent words for *reading* (0·62 and 0·61 respectively: $p < 0·01$). Rates of reading and speaking at the start of treatment were not however predictive of amount of change in disfluencies during speaking. This all means in effect that the higher the rate of reading or speaking at the start of treatment, the greater was likely to be the reduction in reading disfluencies at the end of treatment. Reading again appears to follow somewhat different rules from speaking.

D. SUMMARY

1. Rate of speaking and reading for the group increased significantly over the treatment period, but the group still remained slow when compared with a group of American stutterers. While the two rates of utterance correlated 0·74 at initial testing, their correlation as measures of change was reduced to 0·47.

2. The two measures of disfluency correlated highly at initial testing both for reading and for speaking, but change on one type of task did not correlate significantly with change on the other.
3. Disfluent words and total disfluencies were reduced significantly during treatment. These measures correlated highly and at a very similar level to that found by Sander (1961). In measuring change, however, disfluent words and total disfluencies correlated 0·90 for reading but only 0·59 for speaking. It is possible that this partially reflects fluctuations in interjections, revisions and other normal disfluencies not commonly found in reading.
4. Disfluent word count is a more practical measure for the severe stutterer and it focuses on those disfluencies most commonly diagnosed as "stutters" by the listener. However, more information is gained when both measures are used to assess change. Where differences arise between the two measures for an individual, this can mean he is stuttering less on more words or more on fewer words—a discrepancy can describe a change in stuttering style. If the rate at which words are spoken is added to level of disfluency on these two measures, an even clearer picture is presented of the stuttering pattern of an individual.
5. If a 50% reduction in disfluencies is taken as an indication of significant improvement, 81% of the sixteen stutterers improved significantly on one or both of the disfluency measures; 69% improved on disfluent words alone and 63% on total disfluencies alone. The group changed from being severe stutterers at the start of treatment to being average at the end as compared with American normative data.
6. Follow-up data available on nine of the sample show that:
    (i) one became worse
    (ii) two maintained their improvement
    (iii) two had further slight improvement
    (iv) two definitely continued to improve
    (v) two improved very much more (one a 100%).

III. Interaction Between Speech Disfluency and Implication Grid Measures

A. MEASUREMENT INTERACTIONS

The basic hypothesis for this study was that reductions in speech disfluencies would be related to increase in the meaningfulness of being a nonstutterer. Meaningfulness was operationally defined as the total number of implications in an implications grid.

The hypothesis was supported, both in the case of reduction in disfluent words and in total disfluencies (Sign Test $p < 0.002$ in both cases).

In addition to this, there was a significant correlation between the number of NS implications on the first test occasion and the per cent reduction of disfluent words during spontaneous speech ($r_s = 0.61$; $p < 0.01$). That is, the more the "nonstutterer" construing system was elaborated before the start of treatment, the greater was the chance of a reduction in speech errors. The mean changes on the speech measures and in the number of implications are shown in Fig. 13. The sample numbers on which these mean scores are based range from nineteen on the first occasion to only two on the last.

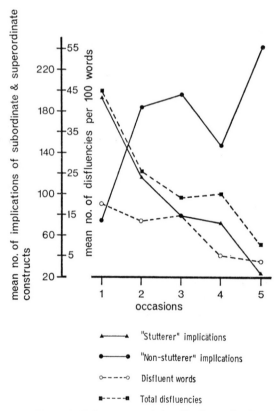

FIG. 13. Mean numbers of disfluencies and implications of subordinate and superordinate constructs on S- and NS-grids on five test occasions.

No predictions had been made about the decline and fall of implications to do with stuttering as the implications to do with fluency increased. It is quite reasonable though that this should be so. The whole reconstruction process is based on the idea of elaborating the stutterer's view of his speech fluency and mention is only made of stuttered speech when it may help to achieve this aim. Construct theory states that we do not have to give up one set of ideas before embarking on the elaboration of another. It is reasonable then to suppose that as one sub-system of constructs becomes more meaningful and is seen to have increasing predictive capacity, the other sub-system will eventually start to "shrivel up" because of its reduced predictive usefulness. Apart from this, the increasing validation of the alternative set of "nonstutterer" constructs and the increasing range of convenience and superordination of these constructs will, almost inevitably, result in the invalidation of some of the implications of the "stutterer" sub-system. However, because of the tremendous individual variability between the stutterers, the speech measures fail to vary significantly with changes in "stutterer" implications over time.

B. IMPROVERS VERSUS NON-IMPROVERS

To step beyond simple addition and subtraction of scores, the group was divided up into two groups: (a) those who had improved more than 50% on either speech measure and (b) those who failed to improve to the level of 50% reduction in disfluencies OR who gave up treatment prematurely for whatever reason even though at time of discharge they may have improved by 50%.

The two groups, "improvers" and "non-improvers", were compared with respect to the *saturation score*. This score represents the extent to which the number of implications an individual sees between constructs approaches the total number that it is possible for him to see. This total number possible is, of course, determined by the number of constructs in the grid.

Taking the grids as a whole, the non-improvers had a significantly higher level of saturation than did the improvers on their S-grids at first testing (Mann-Witney U Test; $p < 0.001$). The two groups did not however differ with regard to the implication saturation on their first NS-grids.

The grids were then divided up into implications of subordinate and superordinate constructs. Looking first at the degree of superordinate construct implication saturation (quadrants c and d in Fig. 11) plotted in Fig. 14, it can be seen that the non-improvers have a far more complex (tighter, more clearly defined, more meaningful) superordinate construing system to do with themselves as stutterers than do the improvers ($p < 0.02$, two-tail test). Figure 15 shows that this does not apply to the non-improvers' superordinate construing of their nonstuttering self *except after several weeks of treatment* when they become differentiated from improvers by consolidating or tightening their system.

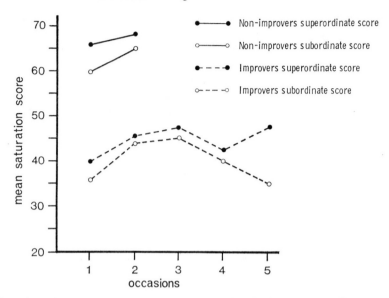

FIG. 14. Mean saturations scores of "stutterer" subordinate and superordinate construct implications for "improvers" on five test occasions and for "non-improvers" on two test occasions.

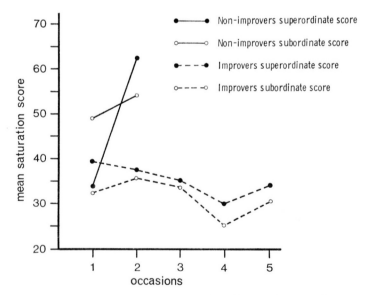

FIG. 15. Mean saturation scores of "nonstutterer" subordinate and superordinate construct implications for "improvers" on five test occasions and for "non-improvers" on two test occasions.

The picture at the subordinate level is almost identical except that the non-improvers have a tighter, or more saturated system to do with themselves both as stutterers *and* as nonstutterers than do those who improve ($p < 0.02$, two-tail test).

To give a clearer impression of what may be going on here, plots of Luke's saturation scores are given in Fig. 16. Luke is an improver who completed six pairs of grids. The sixth occasion was not, in fact, based on newly elicited constructs, but on those elicited for Occasion 5. The sixth test took place after fluency had been fairly consistently established

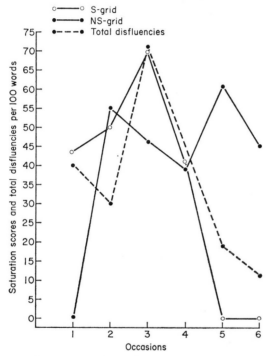

FIG. 16. Total saturation scores on S- and NS-grids and total disfluencies on five test occasions for one stutterer who improved.

and was designed to test the hypothesis that after the sub-system for construing the self as a nonstutterer has become elaborated, the very act of speaking will become increasingly less important. The NS system would not be expected to have a total absence of meaning, since the person would probably tend to equate *me as a stutterer* with *me as a speaker*.

Figure 16 shows the changes that occurred in saturation scores, including the sixth test occasion, on Luke's S- and NS-grids. Because there was hardly any difference between saturation scores at subordinate and superordinate levels, these have been combined and changes on the two types of grid related to disfluency changes.

To be compared with this are the scores for Hilda, the only non-improver to complete more than two pairs of grids. Hilda found speculation about herself very threatening and needed considerable persuasion to undertake it. She was the person who, when forced to write down what she wanted to say (because she could not "get it out") would collect up all the pieces of paper and take them home with her. As a result of helping her to construe herself, she elaborated her NS construing subsystem to some extent—that is, she increased the total number of implications. Then she ceased to attend. Very little change in her speech was apparent, although she ceased having to write things down because of speech blocking.

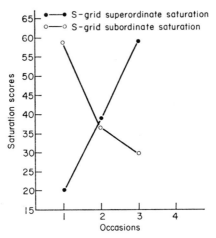

FIG. 17. Superordinate and subordinate saturation scores on S-grids on three test occasions for one stutterer who did not improve.

Figures 17 and 18 show how she tightened her superordinate construing on the S-grid and how her subordinate construing of herself as a stutterer was markedly *reduced* in tightness. On the other hand, both levels of construing tightened on the NS-grids. Could this be a picture one might expect from those who become "happy stutterers"? At a two-year follow-up, she reports being no better or worse, except that she has learned not to mind when she is not able to say what she wants to. If construing at a subordinate level is loosened sufficiently, perhaps this enables one to behave in a way that was previously disconcerting because now, with a looser system, fewer predictions are being made at a "concrete" level. However, this is unlikely since subordinate constructs are assumed to have implications for superordinate construing. More likely, the "nonstutterer" sub-system has elaborated sufficiently for stuttering or fluency to be of equal importance. Stuttering continues because it is the more familiar pattern. This line of argument would lead one to the prediction that had Hilda continued to elaborate her construing of fluency a little further, she would be able to carry out increasingly successful "fluency" experiments.

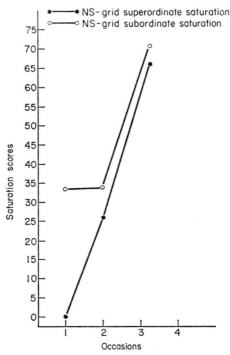

FIG. 18. Superordinate and subordinate saturation scores on NS-grids on three test occasions for one stutterer who did not improve.

No differences between improvers and non-improvers were found in terms of initial severity of stuttering, age, intelligence, neuroticism and so forth. The reason why some failed to improve OR who terminated treatment prematurely (even though they may have reduced their disfluencies by more than 50%) must be sought elsewhere. There are two findings to be considered. One is that those who had more implications to do with being a nonstutterer were more likely to improve. The other is that improvers had initially looser subordinate construct sub-systems to do with being a nonstutterer, suggesting that there may be more bricks but that they are held together with sand rather than cement—the system is more permeable or open to the inclusion of new elements. The improvers also had a "stutterer" sub-system that was less structured.

The "saturation" score has been described as indicating degree of tightness/looseness or permeability/impermeability as if these were synonomous theoretical terms. The score could equally be considered to be a measure of the degree of propositionality/constellatoriness of a sub-system. Particularly so when Hinkle (1965) defines constellatoriness as *the relation between a given construct and others such that a polar position on the given construct implies polar positions on the other constructs* and propositional thinking as that which *implies a suspension of judgment (i.e. a superordinate construction) as to the implicative gain of each of the alternative patterns of construction under consideration.* He suggests that both terms might be looked at as extreme ends of a continuum indicating degree of certainty that particular construct relationships maximize the meaningfulness of the whole construct system (cf. Levy, 1956).

The theoretical tangle can be complicated still further by suggesting that the *saturation score* might more simply be seen as measuring permeability. Hinkle describes a permeable construct as being *one whose range of convenience is relatively unexplored.* He suggests that the total number of implications in the range of implication of a construct might be used as a measure of the meaningfulness of that construct. In this present case, this idea is extended to include construct sub-systems.

Apart from the doubt surrounding the theoretical status of the saturation score, a doubt that will only be resolved by further research, there is reason to think that it may have some practical significance.

C. PROGNOSTIC SIGNS

There are two suggestions that could be followed up by further research. A stutterer seems to stand a better chance of staying the treatment course and of improving if (a) he has a fair number of constructs and implications to do with himself as a nonstutterer to begin with and if (b) he has a sub-system of constructs for construing himself as a stutterer that is relatively permeable and so open to modification (although actual number of constructs to do with *self as stutterer* may not be very relevant). Hinkle (1965) found that superordinacy was related to resistance to change—the more superordinate a construct the more resistant to change it was. From this it can be argued that these non-improvers with more saturated or tightly-knit superordinate *and* subordinate "stutterer" sub-systems, were more likely to resist change.

The non-improvers as a group also seemed to tighten their construct sub-systems further, prematurely (prematurely from the therapist's viewpoint that is) they were indicating that they had had enough. They may have been presented with some evidence that they could construe and, for some reason, have decided that that was enough for the time being. The increase in permeability or tightness of the sub-system could result from perception of threat. Some of their experimenting with the implications of fluency had threatened their remaining system with disruption or radical change. One of the objects of therapy must be to perceive this threat and to try and reduce it and so persuade the person to persevere with his reconstruction of himself in relation to others. It will be noticed that Luke also tightened his stutterer construing sub-system on the third occasion, but was somehow persuaded to continue attending and subsequently to loosen his system again. This process seems to share many similarities with the phenomenon commonly described as "resistance"—the patient effectively "closes shop" on the therapist.

IV. THE PERIODICITY OF IMPROVEMENT

One of the group (Luke) had consistently given ratings throughout his period of treatment. This covered all weeks whether he attended that week or not. He rated his speech on a logarithmic scale ranging from "7" (every word stuttered) to "1" (one word stuttered in every sixty-four). Using this scale, he rated his speech for the best it had been during the previous week, the worst it had been and the average.

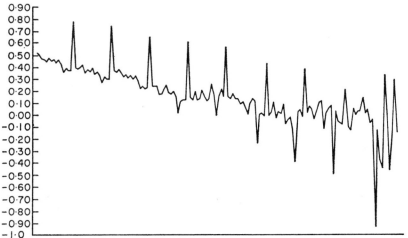

Plot of 150 autocorrelations for the ratings of one stutterer of his 'worst' level of speech during the preceding week

FIG. 19. Set of auto-correlations for 150 self-ratings of the "worst" level of speech experienced during each week by one stutterer.

These ratings were then analysed by the method of autocorrelation (Kendall and Stuart, 1969). This statistical procedure starts out by correlating a set of ratings with itself, obviously producing a coefficient of 1·0. These two identical sets of ratings are then separated by one step, the lower row is moved along one place and another correlation is calculated. The ratings continue to be correlated with each other in this way until there are too few to give a meaningful correlation.

Figures 19 and 20 show how, at intervals of fifteen or sixteen weeks, Luke's ratings of his worst and best fluency level follow a consistent pattern. A look at the raw data indicates that the peaks correspond with the rating of a level of improvement which he had never experienced before. However, this new "good" level of speech was not maintained, he reverted to poorer speech, but not usually to as bad a level as he had had previously. That this pattern of 'two steps forward and one back' became more clear-cut is suggested by the development, in Fig. 19, of a negative as well as a positive peak.

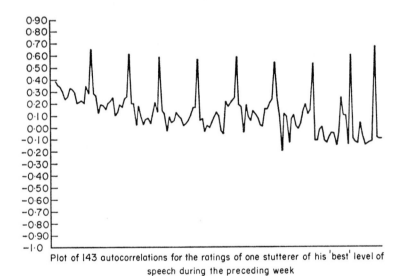

Plot of 143 autocorrelations for the ratings of one stutterer of his 'best' level of speech during the preceding week

Fig. 20. Set of auto-correlations for 143 self-ratings of the "best" level of speech experienced during each week by one stutterer.

The auto-correlations for "average" speech do not show nearly such clear-cut periodicity This could be because to average something, such as one's speech, is psychologically less meaningful than recording the peaks and troughs (See Fig. 21).

This sixteen week or so periodicity is even more striking in its regularity considering it persists irrespective of whether Luke was attending at weekly intervals or not. The fact that he may have been only attending for treatment at three- or four-weekly intervals seems to have had no influence on the pattern.

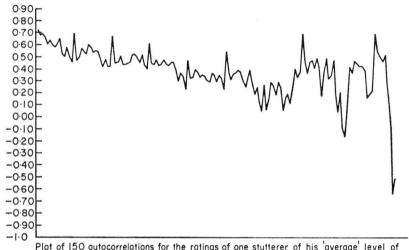

Plot of 150 autocorrelations for the ratings of one stutterer of his 'average' level of speech during the preceding week

FIG. 21. Set of auto-correlations for 150 self-ratings of the "average" level of speech experienced during each week by one stutterer.

This consistent pattern of change seems to suggest that a period of stability is necessary before movement can be started again. It could be that people find it only possible to conduct a limited amount of experimentation at a time and that this has to be followed by a period of reconstruction or consolidation before they can take another step forward again. It also seems, in Luke's case, as if he always tested the limits of experiment to breaking point, the foray always going too deeply into the unknown. When the scene looked too confusing, the threat too great, a degree of retrenchment was necessary. But it was apparently not necessary to go right back, only far enough to make the world a meaningful place again.

It is not possible to relate the changes in speech to specific changes in construing. But there is a suggestion that these new levels of fluency were quite often coincidental in time with the elicitation, laddering or administration of the implications grids. This procedure forces the person to focus on his attitudes in a very concentrated way. It would therefore not be surprising if the whole grid procedure played a prominent part in the reconstruing process. The fact that a person can make use of a technical procedure makes it part of the whole interaction rather than a bit of expertise practiced on the patient by the therapist simply in order to assess him.

The auto-correlations were only carried out on Luke's data, since the ratings were not collected in a sufficiently systematic way from the other stutterers. No conclusions can therefore be drawn from this one demonstration of periodicity of change and only further work will determine whether this is peculiar to this one man or whether similar consistency in change occurs in others, though obviously not necessarily at sixteen-week intervals.

CHAPTER 8

Situation Repertory Grid Analysis

Speaking to your mother is likely to represent many different conditions for different stutterers, or for the same stutterer on different occasions. Even the most elaborately described conditions therefore remain abstractions that subsume innumerable others, and it is impossible either to count them or to make unqualified statements about their effects on stuttering.

A Handbook on Stuttering
O. Bloodstein (1969)

I. STUTTER-FREE SITUATIONS

There can be few more commonly heard statements from adult stutterers than that they are virtually free of their impediment in many situations. This is particularly so when singing, reciting poetry, talking to children, passing the time of day with some pet animal, or when talking to themselves or putting on a foreign accent. Nearly all stutterers have some such series of situations in which they can speak relatively freely. It often seems to boil down to the fact that they are stutter-free whenever they are being other than "themselves" or when the situation does not involve the onus of communicating with other adults. The stutterer who stutters severely when he is talking to himself alone in his room is rare indeed.

In 1949 Bloodstein reviewed the literature concerning the conditions under which the disorder was reduced or eliminated. He found there to be agreement on several social factors that were important, such as the attitude of the listener, the need to make a favourable impression and so forth, as well as the fact that the number of people present to listen to the stutterer speak, makes a considerable difference to the severity with which he will stutter.

Wischner (1950, 1952) considers that there are two types of anxiety relating to the occurrence of stuttering—situational anxiety and specific word anxiety. He cites an experiment (Dixon, 1947) in which stutterers had to read passages of prose in front of one person, five people, and over the telephone. The telephone produced the worst stuttering and the single person audience the least.

Whether it can be concluded that these situations are applicable to all stutterers and whether the list is exhaustive is of particular importance when it comes to carrying out treatment that involves getting the stutterer used to progressively more difficult situations. This is so with the desensitization type of behaviour therapy where emphasis is placed on gradual presentation of a series of situations ordered hierarchically from that least likely to evoke the undesired behaviour to that likely to produce it in its severest form.

In the therapeutic situation one cannot make the assumption that a particular individual will obey the 'situation' rules. Some method has to be adopted to establish which situations elicit stuttering *for him*. This can be done by using a questionnaire or by interviewing. But the therapist then only has a vague idea (if that) as to the equality of the intervals between each situation item in the hierarchy.

The purpose of this part of the research project was two-fold. First, to find out the degree to which stutterers agree on some of the situations likely to evoke their stuttering and, second, to demonstrate a method for establishing, in numerical terms, the size of the intervals between each situation item *for each individual*. The size of the interval may give some idea as to the *degree* of stuttering-potential inherent in the different situations. That is, if situation A has, say, 10 units of stutter-provoking potential, situation B 90 units and situation C 102 units, then more time may need to be spent in desensitizing a person to situation A than B, since the interval between A and B is so large. It may possibly suggest to the therapist that an intermediary situation should be found to reduce the gap.

A. RANK ORDER FORM OF REPERTORY GRID

One of the many forms of grid in current use is that in which the person is required to rank a set of *elements* in terms of certain *constructs*. The elements to be ranked, and the constructs with which to construe the elements, are always chosen in relation to the problem to be investigated. If the problem is the analysis of the individual's construct sub-system concerning cats, then the elements may well be various sorts of cat and the constructs such things as hairiness, temperament, ease of breeding and so forth.

In the present case, the emphasis was on the situations stutterers construe as more or less likely to cause them to stutter. The elements, therefore, concerned talking in certain situations, and the constructs to do with certain expectations a stutterer might have about those situations.

B. THE SITUATION GRID

The elements and constructs used in the Situation Grids were as follows

Elements

1. Talking to a small group of strangers.
2. Talking to a large group of strangers.
3. Talking on the telephone.
4. Talking to women.
5. Talking to men.
6. Talking to my father.
7. Talking to a group of people I know.
8. Talking at a formal discussion.
9. Taking part in an informal discussion.
10. Talking to uncommunicative people.
11. Talking into a microphone of a tape recorder.
12. Talking to people with authority over me.

Constructs

1. Situation in which it is most likely to matter if I make a mistake.
2. Situation in which I am most likely to feel anxious or uneasy.
3. Situation in which I am most likely to stammer
4. Situation in which I am most likely to find it difficult to see or interpret the listener's reactions.
5. Situation in which I am most likely to feel confident.
6. Situation in which I am most likely to resent my stammer.
7. Situation in which I am most likely to expect a critical reaction.
8. Situation in which I am most likely to want to make a good impression.
9. Situation in which I am most likely to want to avoid stammering.

Administration

Cards, on which the element descriptions were written on one side and its number on the other, were placed in front of the stutterer. He was asked to pick out the element best described by the first construct, that is, *the situation in which it is most likely to matter if I make a mistake.* If the subject picked out, say, Situation 12 (*talking to people with authority over me*), he was asked to pick out the next element best described by the construct from the elements minus Situation 12, and so on until all elements were effectively ranked in terms of the *situation in which it is most likely to matter if I make a mistake.*

The element cards were then placed before him again in altered table position and he was asked to construe the elements in terms of the next construct—regarding *anxiety*—and so on, until the same twelve elements had been ranked in terms of all nine constructs (see Table X).

TABLE X

Basic rankings of elements on nine 'situation' constructs by one person.

Constructs	1st	2nd	3rd	4th	5th	Elements 6th	7th	8th	9th	10th	11th	12th
1	12	8	2	1	7	9	6	3	10	4	5	11
2	12	2	1	10	3	8	7	9	5	4	6	11
3	12	8	3	9	2	6	1	7	10	5	4	11
4	10	3	11	2	1	7	12	9	4	5	8	6
5	11	8	9	6	4	5	7	3	2	1	12	10
6	8	12	3	2	1	9	7	10	4	5	6	11
7	8	9	12	7	2	4	1	5	3	6	10	11
8	2	8	12	1	9	3	7	5	10	4	6	11
9	12	8	3	9	2	1	7	4	5	10	6	11

Scoring

The scoring procedure is demonstrated in the analysis of an actual grid. The rankings are entered into a matrix of 9 (constructs) by 12 (elements). The matrix of rankings in Table X now has to be transposed so that each element is described in terms of its rank order. That is, for the first construct, element one was ranked 4th, element two 3rd and so on. The final matrix is given in Table XI.

TABLE XI

Rank order matrix of twelve elements and nine constructs for a 'situation' repertory grid of one person.

Constructs	1	2	3	4	5	Elements 6	7	8	9	10	11	12
1	4	3	8	10	11	7	5	2	6	9	12	1
2	3	2	5	10	9	11	7	6	8	4	12	1
3	7	5	3	11	10	6	8	2	4	9	12	1
4	5	4	2	9	10	12	6	11	8	1	3	7
5	10	9	8	5	6	4	7	2	3	12	1	11
6	5	4	3	9	10	11	7	1	6	8	12	2
7	7	5	9	6	8	10	4	1	2	11	12	3
8	4	1	6	10	8	11	7	2	5	9	12	3
9	6	5	3	8	9	11	7	2	4	10	12	1

The rank order matrix can now either be scored by hand, as described elsewhere (Bannister and Fransella, 1967; Fransella and Adams, 1966), or analysed into its principal components by computer. In this case a special computer programme for analysing grid matrices into their principal components was applied (Slater, 1965).* This programme gives

* These analyses were carried out as part of a Medical Research Council service run by P. Slater.

the intercorrelations between each construct with every other construct and the loadings of all constructs and elements on each component. The loadings enable a pictorial representation to be made of relationships between both constructs and elements. This is only a rough "map" since, for technical reasons, the elements should only be plotted in the "construct space" and the constructs only in the "element space" rather than both together as has been done here. But although there may be statistical reasons for not plotting them together, it is a meaningful procedure psychologically.

Results

A "map" of the grid analysed can be seen in Fig. 22.

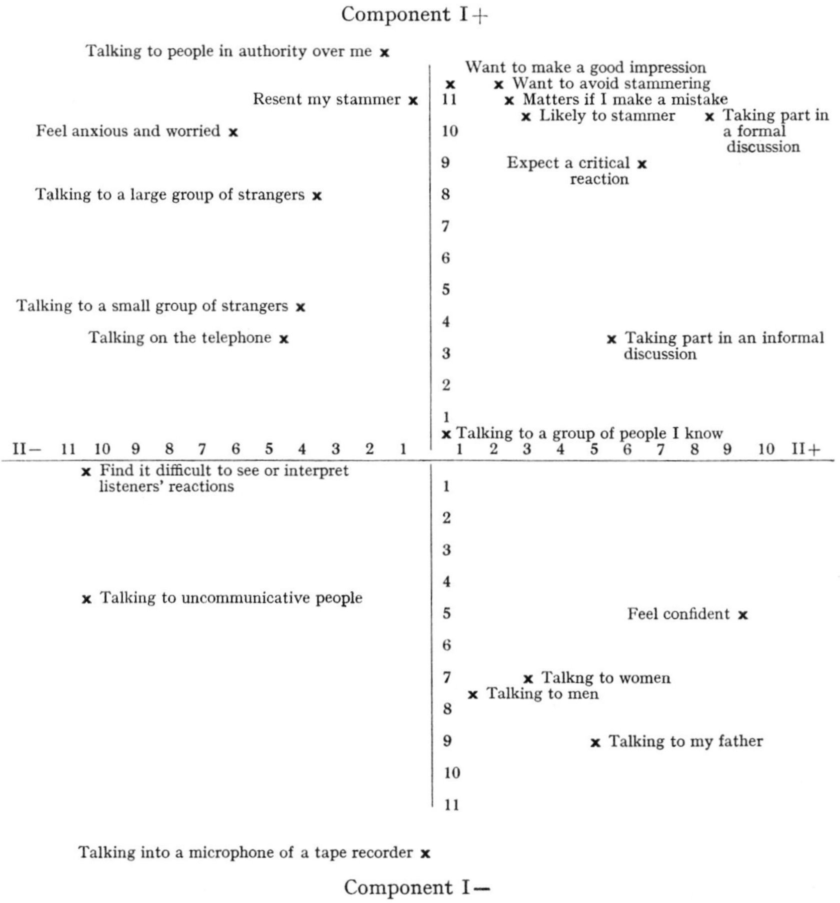

FIG. 22. Plot of construct relationships along two main dimensions of meaning for one stutterer on a "situations" grid.

Apart from this "map", considerable information can be gleaned from the correlations between the constructs. In this form of repertory grid, a correlation can be taken as the operational definition of the degree of similarity–dissimilarity the subject sees between two constructs. For the subject in this example the significant construct intercorrelations were as follows ($r > 0.532$; $n = 12$).

1. *Matters if I make a mistake or am wrong* correlates with:

2. Makes me anxious or uneasy	0·72
3. Makes me stammer	0·81
6. Resent my stammer	0·82
7. Expect a critical reaction	0·74
8. Want to make a good impression	0·85
9. Want to avoid stammering	0·77

2. *Make me anxious or uneasy* correlates with:

1. When I make a mistake or am wrong	0·72
3. When I stammer	0·61
5. When I am confident	0·80
6. When I resent my stammer	0·79
8. When I want to make a good impression	0·80
9. When I want to avoid stammering	0·67

3. *Likely to stammer* correlates with:

1. When I make a mistake or am wrong	0·82
2. When I am anxious or uneasy	0·61
6. When I resent my stammer	0·85
7. When I expect a critical reaction	0·62
8. When I want to make a good impression	0·76
9. When I want to avoid stammering	0·87

4. *Difficult to see or interpret people's reactions* correlates with:
Nil

5. *Likely to feel confident* correlates with:
Nil

6. *Resent my stammer* correlates with:

1. When it matters if I make a mistake or am wrong	0·82
2. When I am anxious or uneasy	0·79
3. When I stammer	0·85
7. When I expect a critical reaction	0·69
8. When I want to make a good impression	0·90
9. When I want to avoid stammering	0·95

7. *Expect a critical reaction* correlates with:

1. Matters if I make a mistake or am wrong	0·74
3. Likely to stammer	0·62
6. Likely to resent my stammer	0·69
8. Want to make a good impression	0·74
9. Want to avoid stammering	0·78

8. *Want to make a good impression* correlates with:

1. It matters if I make a mistake or am wrong	0·85
2. I am anxious or uneasy	0·80
3. I am likely to stammer	0·76
6. I resent my stammer	0·90
7. I expect a critical reaction	0·74
9. I want to avoid stammering	0·86

9. *Want to avoid stammering* correlates with:

1. When it matters if I make a mistake or am wrong	0·77
2. When I am anxious or uneasy	0·67
3. When I stammer	0·87
6. When I resent my stammer	0·95
7. When I expect a critical reaction	0·78
8. When I want to make a good impression	0·86

It was not the object of this study to obtain specific information about individuals and so this grid will not be discussed in any detail, but there is one point worth mentioning. It was extremely unusual in this sample to find Constructs 4 and 5 having no significant correlations with any other construct. In fact, the mean correlation for the group of fourteen subjects between *confident* and *likely to stammer* was -0.804 ($p < 0.001$), and that between *difficult to see or interpret the listener's reactions* and *likely to stammer* was 0.571 ($p < 0.05$). One explanation of this unusual individual finding is that this man was Malaysian. As has been said several times before, because the verbal label is applied to a construct it does not necessarily mean that it has the same implications for everyone, or that it is used in the same way. It is possible that being *confident* and *able to interpret people's reactions* may be irrelevant in Malaysian culture when it comes to construing stuttering and situations relating to it. A similar anomaly occurred in the ratings of two psychiatrists in a group psychotherapy study (Fransella and Joyston-Bechal, 1971; Fransella, 1970b). The British psychiatrist saw the relationship between *scapegoats* and *different from the rest* as being significantly and positively related, while for the non-British psychiatrist the relationship was negative.

Deriving a "stuttering-provoking" score

The aim was to produce a rank order of all the situations according to the extent to which they were perceived as likely to elicit stuttering. The steps in this procedure are as follows.

1. Note down the correlation of each construct with *likely to make me stammer* (Construct 3). N.B. Construct 3 will correlate 1·00 with itself.
2. Square these correlations and multiply by 100 (to remove the decimal point and to make the correlations linearly related).
3. Look to see the ranked position of Element 1 on Construct 1. It is ranked 4th (see rank order matrix on page 148).
4. Divide the correlation squared × 100 (66) by 4 giving a score for Element 1 on Construct 1 of 16·5 (see Table XII).
5. Look to see the ranked position of Element 1 on Construct 2. It is ranked 3rd.
6. Divide the correlation squared × 100 (36) by 3 giving a score for Element 1 on Construct 2 of 12·0.
7. Continue in this way until Element 1 has a score on all constructs and then add all these scores.
8. The stuttering-provoking score for Element 1 is 88·8.
9. Continue in this way for all elements.

For specific details see Tables XII and XIII.

TABLE XII

Details of the derivation of a "stutter-provoking" score from the rank order repertory grid of one stutterer.

	r_s	$r_s^2 \times 100$	1	2	3	4	5	6	7	8	9	10	11	12
1–3	0·81	66	16·5	22·0	8·3	6·6	6·0	9·5	13·2	33·0	11·0	7·3	5·5	66·0
2–3	0·60	36	12·0	18·0	7·2	3·6	4·0	3·3	5·1	6·0	4·5	9·0	3·0	36·0
3–3	1·00	100	14·3	20·0	33·3	9·1	10·0	16·7	12·5	50·0	25·0	11·1	8·3	100·0
4–3	0·15	2	0·4	0·5	1·0	0·2	0·2	0·2	0·3	0·2	0·2	2·0	0·6	0·3
5–3	0·18	3	0·3	0·3	0·4	0·6	0·5	0·8	0·4	0·2	1·0	0·3	3·0	0·3
6–3	0·85	74	14·8	18·5	24·7	8·2	7·4	6·7	10·6	74·0	12·3	9·2	6·2	37·0
7–3	0·62	36	5·1	7·2	4·0	6·0	4·5	3·6	9·0	36·0	18·0	3·3	3·0	12·0
8–3	0·76	58	14·5	58·0	9·7	5·8	7·5	5·3	8·6	29·0	11·6	6·4	4·8	19·3
9–3	0·87	74	12·3	14·8	24·7	9·3	8·2	6·7	10·6	37·0	18·5	7·4	6·2	74·0
	TOTAL		88·8	157·7	110·5	47·8	46·9	50·8	68·9	264·6	99·7	51·4	33·4	343·7

Group results

Having administered and scored the situation grids from fourteen stutterers, correlations between constructs common to all subjects were averaged (z-transformations). Six such constructs were analysed according to their relations with *likely to make me stammer*, and the results are shown in Table XIV.

TABLE XIII

Rank order of elements for likelihood of eliciting stuttering for one stutterer.

	Stutter-provoking score
Talking to people with authority over me	343·7
Taking part in a formal discussion	264·6
Talking to a large group of strangers	157·7
Talking on the telephone	110·5
Taking part in an informal discussion	99·7
Talking to a small group of strangers	88·8
Talking to a group of people I know	68·9
Talking to uncommunicative people	51·4
Talking to my father	50·8
Talking to women	47·8
Talking to men	46·9
Talking into a microphone of a tape recorder	33·4

All the fourteen subjects significantly connected subjective anxiety with likelihood of stuttering, but there was no such high uniformity of construing with any other construct although four of the remaining five had significant mean correlations with the construct concerning likelihood of stuttering.

TABLE XIV

Mean correlations (z-transformation) between the construct *likely to make me stammer* and six other constructs for fourteen stutterers.

Likely to make me stammer vs. Likely to make me anxious to uneasy	0·804···
Likely to feel confident	−0·669··
Likely to resent my stammer	0·551·
Likely to expect a critical reaction	0·515·
Difficult to see or interpret reactions	0·571·
Want to make a good impression	0·380 NS

··· $p < 0.001$
·· $p < 0.01$
· $p < 0.05$

In these grids, as in all other rank order grids, it is useful to build in some rough checks on reliability. For instance, predictions about certain construct relations can be made. In the present example it would have been surprising, and perhaps difficult to interpret, if there had been a non-significant correlation between situations in which the stutter is *resented* and those in which there is a desire to *avoid* stuttering.

The significance levels of 'averaged' correlations are always a problem to assess. In this case, twelve items went into each single correlation and fourteen of these correlations were then averaged. However, statistical significance is not always the same thing as psychological significance and so the more stringent level was taken here, that is, the sample size was taken as fourteen.

As the mean correlations in Table XIV indicate, there was marked similarity in some aspects of construct patterning. Yet some of the differences are also of interest. For instance, one person had no problem with speech as long as the listener knew she stuttered, while another had no problem provided the person did *not* know there was any speech problem. This means that average scores such as these mark interesting, and perhaps important, individual differences.

Discussion

This method for calculating stutter-provoking scores is unusual in that it takes into account the way each situation is viewed across a whole series of construct dimensions. The relationships between likelihood of stuttering and all these dimensions are then summated to give an overall estimate of the stutterer's prediction of stuttering in that particular situation. This is in contrast to the interview method used by many behaviour therapists, where the person is just asked how anxious a particular situation makes him or how likely he is to stutter. The interview method not only does not quantify, it does not get past the simple construct of anxiety or stuttering. It does not take into account the whole cluster of constructs which are used to interpret these situations and which result in the stutterer's prediction of it being a "difficult" or an "easy" situation.

There is no evidence yet available as to the validity of this procedure. It is not known if it reflects *actual* speech fluctuations. However, if subsequent work shows it to reflect severity of stuttering, then it may have value in experimental work not only on determining the relationship between situational factors and stuttering but also in examining the relationships between these situations and other phenomena such as adaptation. It would be interesting, for example, to derive *stutter-provoking* scores for groups of different sizes and with different ratios of men or women. Then, on the basis of these scores, predict the degree of stuttering to be elicited for each stutterer and, possibly, the speed and extent of his adaptation.

As long as stutterers are regarded as belonging to a single group, there will continue to be the large variation attributable to Subjects seen in so much of the experimental literature. The type of procedure suggested might help eliminate some of the Subject variance. In this present very small sample, one subject obtained a *stutter-provoking* score of 83 for talking to women and 177 for talking to men. This was, in fact, the more usual relationship, but for one subject the score for talking to women was 258 and for men 69. For this latter man, talking to women yielded the highest of all his scores. With these two men in a group, considerable difference in the amount of stuttering elicited would be predicted based on the sex of the experimenter alone. In support of this contention is the result of an experiment on conditioning in which the way the experimenter was construed affected the amount of conditioning obtained (Knowles and Purves, 1965).

By focusing on the individual rather than on the group, more might be learned about both situational variability of stuttering and its fluctuation over time.

Section IV

The Treatment

CHAPTER 9

A Description of Personal Change

An essential of successful treatment is the clear realization of the manner in which the stammerer has built round himself a complicated system of psychic reactions which is intended to protect him. To use a metaphor, treatment begins as with the cracking of a nut; the hard shell must be broken before we can penetrate to the kernel. By proceeding too violently, for instance, by using a hammer, we shall spoil the kernel. Even if we use a nutcracker, a tool specially fitted to the purpose, we may still unfortunately do some damage, unless we proceed with reasonable gentleness and delicacy.

Stammering and its Permanent Cure
Alfred Appelt (1911)

It is extraordinarily difficult to give anything like a meaningful word picture of a psychotherapeutic procedure. This is partly because its very essence, the give and take of interaction, is eminently personal to the two parties involved; partly because the theoretical frameworks on which many psychotherapies are based are somewhat nebulous; and partly because the written word cannot convey all the other cues involved in role relationships (in the Kellian sense of one person construing the construction processes of another). There are no non-verbal signs, such as lowering of the head and twinkling of the eye, to help the reader along. To counteract some of these difficulties fairly extensive extracts from the tape recorded interviews of one stutterer are given in this chapter.

A construct theory psychotherapy approach is perhaps slightly easier to convey than many other therapies because it is based on a well elaborated theory. Also, the role of the therapist is clearly defined. With the whole emphasis of the theory being on the person and on the interactions between two construing systems, the therapist does not have to don the guise of the all-knowing seer. Each therapist can "be himself" in relation to the client while following the well sign-posted course of the therapy itself. From the start the client knows that he and the therapist are in the process together and that, if he is lucky, the therapist will help him find a way through the maze of his (the client's) construing in which he has got lost.

After listening to tapes or reading transcripts of the therapy sessions with this present group of stutterers, people have commented that the whole procedure sounds similar to or is *nothing but* behaviour therapy, (e.g. Wolpe, 1958) rational-emotive psychotherapy (Ellis, 1962) or client-centred therapy (Rogers, 1961), occasionally even psychoanalytic therapy.

In this particular approach to the treatment of stuttering, each of these emphases may be seen. There is a considerable use of situations' analysis; the detailing of assignments which the stutterer is supposed to carry out coupled with exhortations to experiment only when he feels all is well, as in some forms of behaviour therapy; there are occasional ding-dong verbal battles to induce the client to "unthink" certain construing inconsistencies and then to act on these new ideas, as in rational-emotive psychotherapy; sometimes there is emphasis on the congruence between the way the person perceives himself and what he is experiencing as in client-centred therapy.

As for psychoanalytic therapy, it has to be remembered that Kelly, when placed in the position of counselling students in the depression of the 1930's, looked to Freudian theory to direct his efforts. He achieved some considerable success with the dynamic approach and, like the scientist he was (having been first trained as an engineer and mathematician), thought he should test the efficacy of the interpretations he gave. He decided to give *any* interpretation that occurred to him *providing* it was likely to seem personally relevant to the client and *providing* it seemed likely to give the client an alternative way of viewing his life. Kelly found that these interpretations were also successful in many cases. It was from this point that he went on to develop his theory of personal constructs and its underlying philosophy of constructive alternativism. Interpretations are therefore sometimes given to the client but here the similarity with Freudian psychotherapy ends. For instance, Kelly considers that much construing goes on unbeknown to the individual. But this is only "unconscious" in the sense that the discriminations he is making are pre-verbal—they have never been verbalized; there is no notion of psychic forces compelling man to action.

A construct theory approach to psychotherapy enables one to use any technique that seems applicable at a particular time with a particular individual, but all are used within one theoretical framework.

This work was primarily undertaken as a research project to show certain relationships between psychological change and stuttering and was not designed to establish the efficacy of a therapeutic process. Therefore there were instances when research intentions dictated one course of action and therapeutic logic another. Topics arising during a session were not pursued if they were not in some clear way related to the theory which stated that stuttering will not diminish until the person construes himself, to some extent at least, as a fluent speaker. For instance, at one point the stutterer started expressing negative feelings toward his father. At the time this occurred, there seemed no way in which this was directly relevant to the research hypothesis, and so it was not followed through.

The description of the therapeutic procedure that follows is presented by giving extensive excerpts of the therapist/stutterer dialogue interspersed with comment. The main purpose being to show the type of changes in construing that occurred and how these related to fluency.

All the excerpts are taken from transcripts of the recordings of the one stutterer. These recordings did not, in fact, start until after the tenth session. There were several reasons for the choice of this particular man to tape record and for not starting at the first session. But the main reason was that it looked as if he would be a very good test of the theory because there was clearly going to be a struggle. He was virtually unable to "loosen" his construing at all. He was twenty-six years old and in many respects a good example of the obsessional scientist—he was interested in fact and not speculation—and he saw the world in these terms. Luke indeed turned out to be a difficult case and had more sessions than any of the others in the sample. He was also the only one of those followed up to relapse after six months without treatment. But, happily, he subsequently wended his way back into the world of fluent people.

In examining the transcripts for examples to demonstrate theoretical points and so forth, it became clear that someone other than the therapist would need to do the same job. I knew the construing system of Luke (as it related to his world of speaking) so well that any analysis done by me was likely to be contaminated by this knowledge. Dr. D. Bannister acted as the independent reader of these eighty-two transcripts.

His views on what he saw in the on-going therapeutic process were compared with my own and only those on which there was agreement are expressed in the comments.

I. From Stuttering to Fluency: A Process of Reconstruction

Before the recordings started, the first S- and NS-grids were completed. As it happened, Luke was unable to provide any constructs for the NS-grid, as he could not visualize himself at all as a nonstutterer. The most significantly related constructs in the S-grid cluster into two groups. There are those relating to the *self* (all evaluatively "good") and those which, at a much higher level of probability, relate to being a *stutterer* (being liked, respected, and ideas about aggression). These *stutterer* constructs occur as persistent themes over the next three years. Lists of the constructs used in each of Luke's grids are given in Appendix 4.

A. THE THERAPY

1st Recorded Session

F. Now, you were going to do some specific tasks, go into shops.

L. Unfortunately, I have only been able to record one.

F. And what happened? What was the situation?

L. I went into a sweet shop and said 'I'll have a packet of Rowntree fruit pastilles please' [laugh]. Yes, because I tried two or three times to do some shopping and it seemed that the things I want were quite involved things and I had to do quite a lot of talking and I stammered doing this and so I determined I'd come a little early tonight and keep buying things until I was successful and luckily I got my tube of fruit pastilles.

F. Describe the scene to me.

L. I went into the shop just outside the front door here and the girl behind the counter looked at me in a sort of questioning way. So I said 'can I have a packet of Rowntree's fruit pastilles please'. So she said 'yes', reached them from the shelf and said 'sixpence please' and so I gave her my sixpence and said 'thank you' and came out.

F. Did you predict you'd say it fluently?

L. Yes, I did, yes.

F. Can you think what made you able to predict?

L. In the first place, fruit pastilles are quite an easy thing to ask for um they were not what I shall call a *status-loaded object*—yes.

F. You'll have to elaborate on that I'm afraid as I don't quite understand.

L. Yes, I've been thinking about the reason why there are some things I find it difficult to ask for and some things I find easy and I have decided that my mind works in this sort of odd way. It attaches to the objects being asked for a certain status; and this status is to do with the showing of my understanding of the object I'm asking for. So, for example, I went into a shop on Saturday to get some wood screws. Now, wood screws come by sizes to which a number is given to the size also by length and also by heads; there are different shaped heads. So there are three things which one must know about wood screws to be able to ask for them directly. Um and so if I go into a shop and ask for number ten wood screws, counter sunk heads, half inch long, then that shows I know what I'm talking about in wood screws. If I say I want wood screws, that shows I don't know what I'm talking about. So um odd isn't it really? So, in knowing all about wood screws and showing I know what I want, I'm able to *command some respect*. Do you know what I mean? Does it make some sort of sense to you?

F. Yes, doesn't it to you?

L. Yes, I think it does, it does make some sort of sense. I think it's fair enough. Um if one wants to show off what one knows and one is able to ask for an object which is classified in a series of different ways and you know how the object is classified you are able to *show off* what you know.

F. Do you think it is just showing off? Couldn't it be that it gives the person something to go on about you? If you ask for wood screws, they wouldn't know if you knew about them or not. By telling them exactly what you want you are telling them that, apart from being intelligent etcetera, you are someone who knows about wood screws. It enables the assistant to put you into a specific slot or category which he couldn't do otherwise. You'd be a nebulous sort of figure. The more nebulous you are I suspect the more likely you are to stutter. Nebulous to the other person that is.

An attempt is being made here to start Luke construing role relationships. Up until now he has done very little construing of other people's construction processes, he looks for concrete evidence that he is respected and if that is not there he has few other ways of weighing up the other person and of adjusting his behaviour on the basis of his constructions of the listener. *But*, as it turned out, I had misconstrued Luke's construction processes.

L. Yes, I don't know actually, because I can't understand why I stammer more when I'm going to ask for something that will enable the person to classify me as a person who knows about wood screws rather than . . .

F. Oh, I'm sorry. Have I got it the wrong way round?

L. Yes.

F. Oh, I thought you stammered *less* when you gave the details.

L. No.

F. I see I beg your pardon—[long pause]. Then you'll have to convince me why it makes sense to you because it fails to make sense to me.

L. Yes. Well, when I said that it made sense to me I meant that it makes sense as far as the effect is concerned, but it doesn't make sense as far as the cause is concerned. See what I mean?

F. No. There seems to be one other explanation, a very simple one. When you ask for wood screws, it demands fewer words than when you ask for wood screws, three inches long, countersunk heads etcetera. Is it anything more than a simplicity–complexity thing?

L. I think it is. I think that whenever I am going to say something which, directly or indirectly will lead me to expect that the other person would respect me or at least that I would get some interest from the other person for saying it, whenever I'm going to say such a thing, my stammer is worse.

Note how the offer of a "simple" technical construction leads Luke to elaborate his construing in order to reject an unacceptable alternative. He was aware that the severity of his stuttering was not simply a matter of the number of words he spoke, but was unable to offer an alternative explanation. I try to help by offering other unacceptable alternatives. By construing what the cause was not he might be helped to construe what it was.

F. I'm a bit foxed at the moment I must confess. Do you want to be respected as a man who knows about wood screws?

L. No [laughs] I think that it is probably the case of anything to be respected for— I want to be respected for *anything*.

F. Normally, respect reduces your stammer doesn't it—in general terms?

L. Yes, yes it does. So what's happening here? I'm going to say something which— and I think to myself 'now when I've said this you are going to respect me for what I've said'.

F. They are going to see that you know something about what they are expert in.

L. Yes, perhaps, yes, yes um and so—now if they respect me and have heard what I've got to say—if they show it's obvious that they respect me and this sort of thing then my stammer will get less. But why does it get bad at first? Why can I . . .

F. In this specific situation, I think this is where the clue must lie. Normally speaking, we've been talking about your work which is important to you. People thinking you are intelligent, have a knowledge of your subject etcetera. Isn't it a bit different going into a shop? Isn't it?

L. Yes. You see, the thing is that I seem to clasp at any opportunity at all to get some respect out of the other person. Now, I can give an example of this between you and I. Do you remember we were talking about how I got this transfer—and that there were two chaps before me and two of them had failed their security check? [Bad stammer on security]. There you see, I don't know if you can remember, but at the time the word 'security' took me a terrific long time. I remember it distinctly. It was in a period of pretty good fluency that blocked absolutely completely and you see here's a thing where a security pass is, at least to some minds, a little bit of *a status symbol*. Again, to the shop keeper here, a chap who knows about wood screws is a bit of a status symbol. Um so, whenever I'm going to say anything—and I think I can generalize this—*whenever I'm going to say anything to anybody which I can regard as a status symbol then my stammer is worse.*

F. And when the respect is genuine, or when you suspect the person respects you for genuine things, then your stammer gets better.

L. Yes.

F. Yes er in other words, you are a bit ashamed going around . . .

L. Yes.

F. Being—is it *big-headed*? Or even—is it even grovelling in a way? Respect at any price?

L. What do you mean?

F. Well, any price being—what I'm trying to get at is that there is a certain amount of almost shame—when one goes about name-dropping . . .

L. Ah yes, that's right!

F. Uncertain of the situation so one says 'Oh well, I must establish my credentials or something, so a couple of names will do it! But in fact, one is a little ashamed at doing it, one should be able to stand on one's own merit.

L. Yes, yes, that sort of thing. Um I um I shall we say, like, not excessively, but I certainly like to—I like the feeling of saying things which are status loaded say, but at the same time I feel that I should be *honest* about it. That's interesting isn't it, I feel I like doing it but I feel I shouldn't.

Here are two examples of the method: (i) the therapist is quite at liberty to say she does not understand, which may be true as in this example, or it may be done deliberately to encourage the client to go on elaborating his construing and (ii) the use of evaluative constructs such as "grovelling" on the therapist's part makes it quite unlike client-centred therapy for example. Again, it is done to help the client find a path through his system, as Luke was eventually able to do to some extent at least. He is verbalizing his ideas about status and finds a major conflict between his desire for status and respect and being "himself" and honest. At the next session Luke explains the outcome of the task set him the previous week, which was to go into a shop and try and buy something *pretending ignorance*. This was to test his prediction that people who are not experts or knowledgeable on a subject are not respected.

Session 2. (Elicitation and laddering of the second S-grid took place during this interview).

F. Did you manage to go into a shop and try and buy something pretending ignorance?

L. No I didn't, because the more I thought about it the more difficult it would be to get exactly the right conditions. Because, what I think is an important aspect of this is that if I went in playing a part I would in fact be acting a role and if you remember, I think we found out some time ago that stammerers could act roles other than themselves and be fluent. So on the basis of this I did not deliberately attempt to do this experiment but of course if a situation should arise in which I *genuinely* found myself in ignorance then I should certainly take note of it.

I did have one situation last week when I was fluent which is an interesting situation, because I had some very strange feelings inside me [laughter].

F. What was the situation?

L. Yes, it sounds odd. I went into this shop and I wanted to buy a quarter pound of sweets or something. I went in and there was a chap serving behind the counter and I imagine that he was the owner of the shop. It was a small sort of shop. Um I said um do you mind if I just look round, I want some sweets, let's see what you've got. Which was quite a fair sentence!

F. That was fluent?

L. Yes, quite fluent. So he said, 'yes, certainly', or something like and er whilst I was looking around he said 'oh, shocking day it's been' and I said 'yes, it certainly has, it makes one wonder where the summer has gone' or something like that. The usual sort of thing one says. And I decided on the sweets that I'd like to have and that was that. The strange thing and the strange feelings were this— as soon as he started to talk I felt that he was a chap who *respected* me [laugh] he sort of—and to my mind he showed that he respected me by the manner in which he talked to me and the way in which he smiled and was as pleasant as he could be and my response to this was almost *a feeling of trying to put him at his ease*. Now, this is a thing I thought was very odd and I tried to put him at his ease in the way I talked back to him so much that I too talked very pleasantly to him. And I felt throughout the entire conversation that I had to be more and more pleasant to him so that I could put him more and more at his ease. How about that! This is a rather odd thing really I thought, because surely a normal person's reaction, if its obvious that somebody respects you, is one of 'oh, well, that's OK, I accept their respect'; whereas I felt a little uncomfortable I suppose in a way, about this chap respecting me and I tried hard to put him at his ease and to try and *make us equal*.

Here is the first clear indication of active role construing. He decides that the shopkeeper respects him and then responds to this construction by trying to "equalize" the situation by putting the man at his ease. The strange *feeling* Luke reports could be the result of several factors. There is the strangeness of the situation itself, he is not used to being aware of so much fluency at one time. There might be some awareness of constructs in transition, and awareness of imminent change. But the most likely explanation is that "putting someone at his ease" is an unusual activity

for him, he is not used to behaving in terms of another person's constructions and it is this that seemed strange or odd. We then go on to look into
this feeling a bit more.

F. Why should you feel peculiar? Because you had not done anything to earn the
    respect of something?
L. No, I don't think it was this. I [pause] I felt uncomfortable that this chap
    should show me so much respect. Now I'm sure that I thought it right and proper
    that he should show me respect. I did not feel that he was such a respect-worthy
    person and I was unworthy of respect or anything like that. I felt that um he
    might not have *liked* respecting me, something like that. So that is to say, I felt,
    rather than myself feeling uncomfortable about the amount of respect being
    given to me, I felt *he* felt uncomfortable about the amount of respect he was
    giving to me.
F. In what way did he indicate this to you?
L. In no way at all. I'm sure that the chap was perfectly happy respecting me.
F. Perhaps he was overdoing it.
L. No, not overdoing it, but probably the amount of respect he showed was
    something that I was not used to—mmmmmmm.
F. That's why you felt uneasy. It was strange.
L. Yes, yes.
F. Why do you think it happened?
L. I don't know, I—all that I said to the chap was 'oh, I wonder if you'd mind if I
    looked around, because I'm not too sure what I want yet', or words to that
    effect and that was all I said. So his impression or his attitude had to be based
    solely on that and my personal appearance and what I said to him and immedi-
    ately he sort of said, 'certainly, please do' and all this sort of thing, *extremely
    courteous in the way that I would be to anyone I respected.*
F. You did him the courtesy of saying 'do you mind if I look around', didn't you?
L. Yes.
F. I mean, a lot of people go into a shop and pay no attention to the person at all
    don't they?
L. I don't know.
F. They just look around. But you'd acknowledged his presence and I don't see
    anything surprising in his response.
L. No, no I don't really see anything surprising. I think the main thing that is
    surprising is my attitude.
F. Yes.
L. My feeling that I had to even things out.

In this interview there is again the idea of *status* in his attempts to
"equalize" the relative positions. He continues to elaborate his construing of respect in role terms and his response to this. One way of showing
respect is to be courteous, but he sets limitations on this role construing
by making it self-referent; 'he was as courteous to me as I would be to
someone I respected'. However, right at the beginning of the session he
explains how he cannot deliberately role play a situation, but has to wait
for it to "genuinely" arise. These themes of *respect, status* and *honesty* or

genuineness recur over and over again up to and including the last interview.

At the next session, during the elicitation of constructs for the second NS-grid, several apparently "new" constructs emerged, such as *suave*, representing a steady elaboration. But these new constructs are still very closely linked with the central *respected* versus *no respect* (now *common*) construction, as if he were examining the network around a central point once it has been discovered. Of some significance is the giving of *common* as the opposite of being *worthy of respect*.

Session 4

After an incident of complete fluency talking to friends.

F. This was a very unusual experience, what thoughts went through your mind? Obviously you watched yourself with some interest.

L. Yes. I found that the more I realized that I was talking fluently the more I relaxed and the more the feeling of confidence came on and the feeling got better and better.

F. Did it give you any new insights into the fluent "you" that is going to be?

L. I don't think so because I think that I have always been aware what the "fluent me" is.

Later extracts show in fact, how impoverished are his ideas about the "fluent me" and how these gradually become clarified. We continue to discuss this episode further.

L. My wife and I were visiting my friend from work, and his wife. We had a great long talk, he and I basically. A discussion about something and the other two joined in. It was quite a long discussion. I was expounding my views most eloquently. I—this was the best that my wife has ever heard me.

F. In company.

L. Yes, actually or even where she alone is concerned. She remarked on it afterwards. It gave her an insight into what I would be like.

F. Did she like the insight?

L. She was very impressed [laugh]

F. What did she say?

L. She thought that I was far cleverer than she had previously thought. [laughs]

F. That was very nice.

L. I was quite pleased really. The thing is really that whenever I enter a discussion and want to get over something that has a lot of information in it I usually stammer pretty badly. But we were talking about something that is one of my pet subjects and I was waxing quite eloquent and I was quite surprised.

We now come to the laddering of the constructs elicited from the second NS-grid the previous week, starting with *worthy of respect— common*.

F. So we come to *worthy of respect versus common*. Now, being worthy of respect is presumably preferable to being seen as common, the question is why, for you, is it preferable?

L. Well, the only thing I can say is that *common* people are *not respected*, but that's not much of an answer is it. Er . . .

F. No, it goes in a bit of a circle, doesn't it?

L. Yes, it does. I think that *commonness* is associated with *ignorance* and *worthy of respect* is associated with *intelligence*. I think that *common* people have *no status* and *people with respect* have *status*.

F. That is, people worthy of respect?

L. Yes, yes, have status, common people have not.

F. Now that we have got on to the status one, why does one want status?

L. I tend to say to myself I want status but never asked myself why. Yes, I think it's basically because when you have status people respect you and this sort of thing and the way they show this is by being eager to please you. That is to say, because they are eager to please you they will do things for you and help you without arguing about it or in fact without refusing to do it.

F. Can you sum that up?

L. People are more helpful to a person they respect.

F. Now, a person who has status—are these equated terms, respect and status?

L. Ah, I see what you are getting at. In my mind they are. I think that people want to impress other people who have more status than they have and they impress them by being nice to them. I can well imagine that I would want people to be nice to me because I wouldn't know what to do if they were nasty to me. I think that we are actually coming on to this when we get to *aggressive* versus *gentle*. I think that this is actually something we have missed out. I think that this aggressive versus gentle is as important as respect.

F. No we've never had it before. Now, I have just got down here 'command help from others'. Would that be right? In other words, people who have status like this because they command help and friendliness and all these other things from others?

L. Yes, I think the main point is that people who have *status* are *less likely to be refused*.

F. Whereas people who do not have status are more likely to be refused.

L. I—don't think I could necessarily handle—no, would know how to get a person to change his mind.

F. That's an interesting idea, isn't it? In a way, it puts the status idea into place because it becomes understandable now, doesn't it?

L. Yes.

F. It has always been a very strange idea to me. It has obviously played a great part in everything.

L. It may have been a strange idea to you . . .

F. By strange I mean it was difficult to see why it played such a large part.

L. Well, I think that this is the thing. If one has status or is respected, which is the same thing, then if someone is infinitely respected they would say what they want to a person who would immediately rush off and do it. If a person commanded zero respect and they said to someone I want so and so, their reply would be 'go and do it yourself'. And so as everybody lies somewhere between these two—but I suppose the majority of people would be happy about having people refuse to help them or having people downright rude to them.

F. Oh, come off it! I certainly don't!

L. Well, you'd—I think you'd probably be able to sum up the situation and sort of say something that made them change their mind, wouldn't you?

Here is an interesting example of the discovery of what seems like an implicit pole. Luke has been talking about respect commanding help from others and then comes on to the question of people being nasty to him, i.e. lack of respect inviting aggression from others.

This rather extraordinary belief in the social competence of 'the majority of people' was challenged by me in a forthright manner and I went on to give an example of a situation in which I had been nonplussed. This had the desired effect of making him put the idea into words:

F. I don't think that you can assume that everyone can deal with these situations automatically and that it is only you who can't. It is not necessarily only to do with speech.

L. That is a very interesting thing that, because I feel that *fluent speakers can deal with any situation and that if I was fluent I would be able to do it.*

F. I don't think this is necessarily so. No.

L. [a sound of surprise]. A lot of this will be of importance I think later on when we come to the aggression idea.

This is a really remarkable revelation of the narrowness of the range of convenience of the fluency construct. He feels that fluent speakers can deal with any situation, indicating how completely his interpretation of interpersonal relationships has been related to, and understood within, the compass of his stuttering. Hence his surprise at the existence of all kinds of interpersonal prediction and understanding problems right outside the question of stuttering and fluency. It can be seen as a startling illustration of how superordinate the construct *stuttering versus fluency* is in his construing system. The session continues with a discussion of the aggression–gentle construct.

F. Well, we have just got there. Let's have a look at it. *Aggressive* versus *gentle.* Which would you prefer to be seen as, or prefer to be?

L. I don't know. I imagine that the person who—I imagine that a fluent speaker with my personality would say *gentle*, but I think that in my present state I would rather be seen as *aggressive*. Um. Where does one start? I suddenly became aware of a feeling that I would not know what to do if somebody was aggressive towards me and so it would be very nice if nobody was ever aggressive towards me. That is to say, my personality to other people seemed to be an aggressive one and I frightened people so much that they wouldn't dare to be aggressive towards me—um—I very foolishly—and yet it is there—I feel very concerned when I pass aggressive-looking people in the street.

F. Concerned in what way?

L. Concerned lest they should become aggressive towards me and I should not know what to do. I don't know if this happens. Aggressive young men, going around in gangs of four or five. I heard that they obstruct the way and push people off the pavement and things like that. I am always very apprehensive when passing aggressive-looking young men lest they should do this to me. This hasn't happened—but . . .

F. Why do you think this is so?

L. I am concerned lest I should not know what to do. I wouldn't know whether to try and box them about the ears or whether to just walk on and try to ignore it.

F. Do you think this has got anything to do with the fact that you stammer?

L. I can imagine it might have. One thing which I am looking for in the cause of my stammer is a clue that the cause must be a thing that has remained practically unchanged since the age of four years old onwards. This desire for respect cannot have existed at the age of four and there is something wrong here I feel . . .

F. Well, it could be the result of stammering.

L. Yes, it *could* be.

F. I suspect that the wanting of respect stems from the stammer rather than the stammer from wanting respect.

L. This may be so, but I do not immediately feel that this is so. I still feel that I am under-respected.

F. We glibly say that children do not want respect. Could we be wrong in this?

L. Yes, we could indeed be wrong. Yes—we—I think we are wrong. I used to play with the squire's son so to speak, who was about the same age as I was. I can remember the case of going into a shop and we both ask for a pennyworth of sweets. With the squire's son there was a great deal of rubbing of hands and nothing was too much trouble, whereas with me it was 'what do *you* want?' So I think we are probably underestimating the importance of this. But again, I'm sure that the majority of people do not go around being afraid they will be pushed off the pavement or something like that.

F. It is difficult for me to say because I think women would feel differently from men. They would have a right to feel apprehensive. I was wondering about stammering—you wouldn't be able to fight them verbally which is the obvious thing to do.

L. Yes, I agree. I think in a situation such as this I would draw upon my special fluent reserve that I keep for emergencies and I wouldn't stammer, but I certainly wouldn't know what to say. I wouldn't know how to bring somebody down to size. The only sort of means of defence I have would be purely a physical one.

F. But are you sure you are the only one who feels this? I would hazard a guess that if you were to ask a lot of men you . . .

L. I think that not with the frequency that I fear it, no. You see also—ah, yes, something else. Also connected with this is again a *status* thing. These young men that I'm afraid of *resent my status* and er, that is the reason why they are aggressive to me, not because I am weaker, but because I'm better than they are. Also, of course, there is the situation where there's no fear of physical violence to myself, but you get young lads of about ten or twelve or so. If I take my wife out for a walk they're running about and mucking about together probably swearing or using very bad language. I think this is very wrong because extremely bad language is unnecessary and it's also offensive to other people. I'm sure it must be offensive to my wife and I feel that I would like to be able to verbally say something to these youngsters to put them in their place or something like that, er even if I was fluent I wouldn't know what to say, er I don't even know whether I'd be justified in saying anything, I feel that I should, out of respect for my wife and also out of my own offended sense of what was right. Er, I certainly wouldn't say anything if I were by myself. I suppose that my wife is the deciding factor. Um, again I feel at a loss in this situation. This situation makes me feel very uncomfortable because (a) I stammer but (b) *if I didn't stammer I still wouldn't know what to say to these young people to put them in their place.* Here again is something which is tied up with aggression. If I had an aggressive personality, if I looked aggressive, I could say to these youngsters 'how dare you use such language' and they would slink away suitably frightened. If I said it looking gentle, like I am, they would say 'you so-and-so' which would offend me even more and make me look rather ridiculous in front of my wife. So again, here is an example of not physical aggression but fear of verbal aggression.

When he talks about the possibility of young boys annoying his wife while they are out and says he would not know what to do about it *even if he were fluent,* he seems to be exploring again the newly discovered possibility of problems of interpersonal interaction which are quite independent of the question of stuttering. This is also another example of the relative meaninglessness to him of being a fluent person as opposed to being a stutterer. I continued by encouraging him to think about fluency in relation to coping with aggression—toned down to 'off-hand replies'. Before very long this becomes linked into the status/respect network.

L. Yes, I do get off-hand replies now, but it is from people of my own status, and I'm quite happy with them. If I thought a well-educated chap was going to push me off the pavement I would be perfectly happy to give him a punch on the nose. I'd be perfectly happy about this, but if a rough labouring chap did that I'd be frightened.

F. I see. You wouldn't say to yourself 'oh, well, he doesn't know any better' or something?

L. No. I wonder. I'm not certain of this, but I wonder if my dignity would be offended. 'How dare he, *common*'—sounds terribly snobbish doesn't it—'how dare he, a common person, dare to attempt to push me off the pavement'. I'm—I think that dignity must come into this.

F. But if you say to yourself 'he doesn't know any better', isn't it like the thing we discussed a while ago, about people not paying attention to what you are saying or—yes, what you are saying? Now most stammerers get a bit het-up about this, they stammer more if they get an off-hand reply. There is the immediate awareness that a great many people do not care twopence about them, and are not going to listen to what they say and so on and this is one of the things they have got to come to terms with, half the world doesn't care about them. Most stammerers, and I don't think you are any exception, live in a very egocentric world, it revolves around them much more than it does around most other people, because of their stammer, because they have been used to being the centre of attention, because they are unusual. Therefore, you think that anyone who pushes you off the pavement, that this is directed at you *as a person.*

L. Yes, I see.

F. It has probably never occurred to them, you are just in their way, you know, an object in their way.

L. [large sigh] Yes, I feel that people who are not respected resent people who are respected. And the people who are not respected are liable to show their resentment in the form of aggression. If I went out in a dirty pair of gardening clothes or jeans and a shirt or something like that, I would step along the pavements perfectly confident. I'd have no apprehensions at all. Because, as far as the common people are concerned, I am also a common person and I would fear no aggression from them.

F. Supposing one of them pushed you off the pavement?

L. I do not imagine that this would happen. In the unlikely event of this happening, I should catch hold of him and throw him off the pavement. Very funny this. I'm sure there is something wrong here you know. If I go out dressed in a very smart suit with my white shirt on and my tie neatly knotted and shoes gleaming, shining, and I see a person in jeans coming towards me, I feel that this person resents me and is liable to show his resentment in the form of aggression. Something definitely wrong here isn't there? I'm sure that this is an important factor in my stammer. I can't really place why, I can't place a specific instance in my life which has led to this.

Luke's assertion that he would know what to do if he were pushed off the pavement by a well-dressed "respected" person but not if it were a scruffy common sort of person, and then his attempt to construe this as demonstrating a lack of respect for him on the part of the common person, could mean that this umbrella term *respect* here is really a synonym for *understanding*. That is, Luke's difficulty is that he can't construe such people and therefore doesn't know why they would push him off the pavement or what they would be likely to do next, or how they would react to whatever he might do. Similarly, he feels that *they* would have no appreciation or understanding of *him*. At the present time he has very little in the way of constructs to choose from and tends to see everything in terms of *respected–common*. He was not prepared to accept the attempt on my part to limit the range of convenience of this construct, by suggesting that some people just may not pay attention to him.

Right at the end of this important session, almost as he was about to leave, he gave an interpretation of the *common–aggression* situation bringing out very clearly the importance of the construct *genuine–pretending*, which is to play an increasingly important part in the months to come. Dressed in jeans he is being *genuine*, but dressed in a smart suit he is *pretending to be something he is not*.

L. I believe that common people do not resent me because I have status, but rather common people resent me because they see me as another common person who is—what's the word?

F. Putting-on? Assuming?

L. Yes, pretending to have status or assuming to have status which doesn't belong to him.

Soon after this there comes a good example of the use that is made of the role relationships within the sessions themselves. Luke construes the therapeutic role relationships in connection with his stutter thus.

L. I definitely think this point you made is important about the majority of people being unable to handle aggression in [severe stutter] in all situations.
F. That was a very good example of a "7" stammer.
L. Yes, it was, yes. I can tell you the reason for it as well!
F. Yes?
L. [laughs] I can well believe that er this um I can well believe that this er aggression of mine is sufficiently maladjusted for you to lose respect, self-respect, for me!
F. I see.
L. So that's the reason for that. There's a weighing up going on in the mind as to how much respect I will have lost because of the maladjustment of my aggression. I think. So you will see that respect is important.

Session 5

This starts off with Luke's problem of how to predict the reaction of an assistant at work if he were asked to do something. The whole issue again centres around the idea of whether people respect him or how he can deal with people who are not like him. But since he has only a fairly concrete perception of people, he measures 'being like me', or the degree to which people are 'like me', on a very simple direct measure in terms of dress.

I start off by challenging his views with a very simple logical notion of evidence (i.e. if people have always obeyed one in a situation, then that is proof positive that there is no need to worry about them not obeying) in an attempt to find out what he uses as validating evidence for his construction of respect and relative status. In trying to explain what is unsatisfactory about this view, it rapidly becomes obvious that what Luke means is that you do not know what significance the assistant attaches to the whole situation regardless of the fact of whether he helped you out or not. In other words, the unknown that always keeps the situations in doubt, is not the actual *behaviour* of the other person, but his possible *attitude* towards the whole incident.

Once again I try hard to limit the range of convenience of the constructs used so that he will not try and draw from simple job interactions implications of great core role significance. Note how he insists that the assistant might think 'who does he think he is' if Luke gives him orders. This is really saddling the assistant with the key question of Luke's life.

We approach the topic by discussing the various ways in which one can ask someone to do something.

F. This is interesting isn't it, because in the past you have had only one way to ask something—to stammer.
L. Yes
F Is that right—really?

L. Well, yes, but as far as I'm concerned there are still different ways of asking—in actual words—the actual context of my sentence.

F. Yes, but don't you think that when you ask somebody something, like an assistant at work, he will only see you as a stammerer and the words you say, you may try to say them in a different way, but what comes over is the same.

L. Yes, yes, this is probably true um but er until recently I thought that people didn't really see me as a stammerer.

F. No, you didn't think it consciously. No. But the feeling must have been there surely.

L. Probably. Yes, probably. Yes. Now today, I did ask an assistant to give me some help. We were doing something and I asked him without stammering. But I was still unable to judge what his reactions would be. Indeed, I was unable to judge what his reaction was *afterwards*.

F. Did he do what you wanted?

L. Oh, yes. That's the most important thing.

F. Why do you doubt that he was quite willing to do it?

L. This is er something which I am always on the guard against. So in every situation, because I am on guard, I naturally doubt whether the person actually will or won't.

F. But one does work on evidence, do we agree?

L. er um . . .

F. Let me put it this way. If you never saw a sign of anybody doing something for you unwillingly, you surely would start to accept that there was not anything there to see.

L. Yes, when it is said like that it sounds logical. But I think that I have tended to approach every situation, or every situation when I want someone to do something um—tended to regard that situation as completely a new situation.

F. Yes. You haven't added them up and looked at the probabilities overall.

L. No.

F. I wonder if this is because for every stammerer each situation *is* a new one in a way. Because you can never be quite sure how badly you are going to stammer.

L. Could be, yes. Um or it could be because he is never quite sure how the previous situation turned out.

F. He is in constant doubt either way.

L. Yes.

F. Whereas a fluent speaker of course isn't.

L. No.

F. For him the situations are additive, aren't they?

L. Yes. You see, if I went into a garage and said 'could I have three gallons please', I wouldn't doubt that the attendant would give or would not give me petrol. But if one asks someone to do something I would doubt that. I think probably with the petrol-pump attendant the role is sharply defined. He is there to give you petrol. But an assistant is also there to assist one. No, I think that also with the petrol pump attendant you don't really care what he thinks of you.

F. It is a temporary relationship.

L. Yes, it is a temporary relationship, an assistant's permanent and so um whenever I ask an assistant to do something, I wonder to myself 'now is he going to think afterwards 'oh, *who does that chap think he is asking me to do things*'!

F. You can never prove the contrary to yourself can you as long as you are looking for negative evidence. You are not looking for positive evidence are you?

L. I don't know. I think I am probably looking for positive evidence. The evidence whereby he says 'I consider it perfectly right that I should help you'.

F. How do you think a person would show he was willing to help you? How would you behave if someone asked you to help them?

L. I'd say, 'yes, certainly'.

F. How would they know that you were quite willing to do it?

L. Because I'd say 'yes certainly' and help them to the utmost of my ability and afterwards when they said 'thank you', I'd say 'that's perfectly all right'.

F. How do these people behave to you when you ask them to assist you?

L. They say 'all right', which is not the same as 'certainly'.

F. Wouldn't you say 'certainly' more to an equal? If I said to you 'would you help me please', you'd say 'certainly'. If I were to say to a student 'oh, come and do these figures for me will you please', I wouldn't expect them to say 'certainly'.

L. Wouldn't you? [very surprised]

F. No. Why should they? They probably don't want to do the wretched figures anyway, but they do them because they know I have the right to ask them. They may hate figures.

L. Um I see. [deep sigh] You see, I think that this is what's wrong with me to a certain extent. Um O.K. So I've got the right to ask. But I would like to think that I would be helped even if he was not an equal or, well, say I'd like to get away with it on the basis of my personality alone or something like that.

F. But you are asking too much, aren't you? Because this is not the role relationship, is it?

L. I see. [deep sigh] No.

F. If you were outside and your car had broken down and the same assistant came along and you said 'oh, could you help me?' he might then say 'certainly', because now you would be on an equal footing.

L. I see, these are things which have completely escaped my comprehension.

F. The status is in the job not the person. If the person is nice so much the better.

L. I see. So if then I asked an assistant to do something and he said 'no, I can't, I'm busy doing something else', then I'm stumped.

F. What could you do?

L. I'd like to say, 'well just leave it for a few minutes and help me', but I wouldn't because I feel I might in doing that be over-stepping the mark and the assistant would think 'who does he think he is ordering me about!'

Shortly after there came a clear illustration of the kind of dilemma Luke makes for himself when he indicates that either end of the construct *pleasant–firm* can result in *lack of respect*.

L. Can a person be too pleasant? If I went around asking everybody in very polite language, would they think 'well, that chap isn't very sure of himself!?'

F. This is one way of showing it, isn't it? Not being sure of oneself?

L. Yes, yes.

F. Not being sure of your particular role in that situation. A person who is sure would be *pleasant* but *firm*, he shows what he wants, what he expects.

L. Yes. I would rather be pleasant and firm than just pleasant.

F. Oh, surely they have got to go together, haven't they? For anyone who is in charge of people?

L. They should, yes. So, how firm should one be? I mean to say if one is extremely firm, people say 'oh, crikey, he's a firm sort of chap' and are not very keen on his attitude.

F. Surely it's a case of if you go and ask someone—that is the fluent you—you put it in a very nice way, but with the feeling behind it that you expect they will do what you are asking. Rather than begging them to do it.

L. Yes, yes. You can see what I am up against. *Just knowing how far to go with things before I become objectionable.* Take for example the *soft-firm* axis, or whatever you call it. If you are soft, people say 'well, that chap isn't very sure of himself' and they lose respect for you. If you are extremely firm they say 'oh, he's a hard sort of chap' and lose respect for you. So at either end of the axis is a case where respect is lost. Somewhere there is maximum respect. Where I find it difficult is where I only have a very shaky idea of where that maximum respect would come.

This idea of how extreme you can be with certain types of behaviour is also a constant theme and played a large part in the temporary relapse that followed six months after the end of treatment. In elaborating construing of himself as a fluent person he is encouraged not only to explore the implications but to experiment. In this case evidence alone will show him how far he can go in being firm without being objectionable. His relapse almost three years later occurred when he found he did not like the aggressive person he had become.

Session 6

In a discussion about the periods of fluency that had occurred since the last session, Luke talks about forgetting how it "feels to be fluent" when he is stuttering.

L. I don't forget completely, I can remember that during the afternoon say, the previous day, I was very fluent, but now, when I'm speaking to you, I cannot remember what it felt like. Actually, as a matter of fact, as I was saying that very sentence, this feeling has come back again and I've begun to remember what it is like.

F. Was that because the previous sentence came out very well indeed?

L. No, the preceding sentences came out pretty well because at that time I remembered and my fluency started immediately from then. It's the oddest thing, isn't it? It's just as if you turn a switch or something like that.

* * *

F. When you say forget, you know intellectually that you can speak fluently but you forget the feeling, is that it?

L. Yes. Um I suppose so. I think there's probably a difference between believing something intellectually and believing something and believing you are actually or have actually done something, do you know what I mean?

This distinction between believing something intellectually and "feeling" it has occurred before can possibly be considered an example of a man wrestling with his own hostility, in the Kellian sense. He is aware of invalidation of his construing but cannot as yet accept the implications.

This occurs again more clearly in the next excerpt in which there is a long discussion about what people think of him in certain situations.

F. Why should they suddenly turn round then and say 'oh, he's a standoffish so-and-so who pays no attention to our jokes?'

L. I suppose I have often listened to other people saying 'oh, so-and-so he's a standoffish chap, he cut me dead' and I suppose I mentally made a note 'do not cut people dead'.

F. But we are not discussing cutting people dead.

L. No, but I suppose that I have probably clocked up so many of these sort of things like cutting people dead, not listening to jokes and so on, everything in which a person has said *'who does he think he is'* sort of thing. Any situation whereby a person's character has been criticized for some aspect of this respect sort of thing or of forcing one's authority upon somebody, or ordering people about, bossing them, any situation like this I have mentally clocked it up and said 'I mustn't be like this' and so I've got a whole list of things which I mustn't be like.

F. But you have not got anything which tells you what you *should* be like.

L. No. Well I suppose that I can be *anything* providing I'm not like this. I suppose I see every person as someone who is going to judge me for something.

F. I suppose that people always do judge stammerers don't they. I mean, this is an enormous judgement 'he is a stammerer' for a start. They never take you as a person, do they? They never have done all your life. They make a judgement right from the start. But now with fluency you are expecting the same quantity of judgements. They're not going to be there.

L. Yes.

F. By and large, we take people as they come. A person's pleasant and intelligent and is accepted at his face value as an intelligent, pleasant person.

L. Um I can feel inside me that this is a pretty big obstacle to get over. You know I listen to what you have to say and I, intellectually shall I say, I agree with it. But as soon as I try to get my mind to accept it, it comes up against a brick wall.

F. Oh, yes. I don't think this will come easily at all. But the more incidents you build up in which nothing disastrous happens . . .

L. Because it is always difficult to tell if anything disastrous has happened—in a given context. Because after all, if someone thinks you're a bit bossy, say, they are not going to say it to your face, are they?

This last comment shows Kellian *hostility*, a true tampering with the evidence. He is saying that *his* construing of other people's reactions must stand, even though there is no evidence that the construing is accurate. It is necessary for him to be hostile here because important aspects of his construing are being threatened (awareness of imminent comprehensive change in one's core structures). If he accepts the invalidations I am offering he has no alternative constructs with which to replace them—he is faced with chaos.

Session 7

In this session there is evidence of very conscious core role construing in the distinction being made between the 'old' versus the 'new' self.

F. Have you done any more observing or thinking about dealing with assistants? About being firm?

L. I did actually. I asked an assistant to do things for me. There was a great temptation for me to fall into the routine of being over polite and that sort of thing, but I more or less rehearsed what I would say in just an ordinary 'oh, would you mind helping me if you can spare five minutes' and this is what I said. And because it was of some importance, you know what I mean, I stammered quite a bit on it. It was rather unfortunate, but it worked. He said, 'all right'. Still—it still tends to feel a little odd. It isn't the old me, but it is definitely the me that is there.

F. Did he give any indication that he thought badly of you?

L. No. In fact I—if I thought anything about it—I probably thought he thought this chap is behaving a little more like a natural person.

Session 8

There is an indication now of progress in restricting the overall use of the construct *respect*.

L. I was saying that I am pretty confident now that I know in what way people are summing me up, and with a stranger it is usually not very important to me how they sum me up. Certainly, strangers wouldn't see one at the depth that one's friends would sum you up. Therefore, I can't really understand why my speech should be so bad with them.

F. Well, I wonder. Last week I think you said that you did not know people were intelligent until you talked to them, so friends can get at this information whereas a stranger can't.

L. I would not necessarily want strangers to sum me up like this.

F. What other ways are they going to sum you up in?

L. What I mean is, I meet a stranger, and this chap says 'oh, this chap is a stranger to me I'm not going to bother to meet him again, I won't have to go through all the rigmarole of summing up this character'.

F. But you've said before that you want respect from everybody.

L. Yes. I've changed my mind. There are some people who are ships that pass in the night, that I'm not bothered about.

At the same time as restricting the range of convenience of the construct *respect* he added a new implication.

L. Whereas I've in the past probably been looking for people to respect me because of my class or position, what one really needs is for people to respect one for being a *nice chap*.

The reconstruing occurring during this and the previous week has lead to an improvement in both "worst" and "average" ratings.

Session 9

Luke's speech has changed to the extent that the subject of stuttering rather than fluency tends to be discussed more and more. Stuttering becomes more and more the exception that has to be accounted for.

There is still, however, great poverty of ideas about personal interaction and considerable naïveté in interpersonal construing. Also, at this stage Luke has virtually nothing to say on the very important idea of experimenting with voice expression, hand gesture and so on. He sees these things as only being relevant in relation to stuttering.

Session 10

Although there has been considerable overall improvement in the amount of fluency and some movement in construing, the following statement indicates that, in core role terms, Luke still views himself very much as a stutterer. This gives us some insight into the rather wild fluctuation in ratings over the previous three weeks.

F. Do you know when you are going to stammer?
L. I think I do—I think there is a feeling almost that *I am a stammerer* and therefore that I should stammer.
F. It's an idea.
L. Well no. It isn't in this context alone—it's in every sort of situation. I—as a matter of fact, this was something that I was waiting for an opportunity to mention. Even now, at this very instant when I'm talking pretty fluently—I have been for about five minutes—I feel it's wrong—I can feel this in me. I feel I'm talking fluently but I shouldn't be.
F. Can you analyse it? In what way does it seem wrong?
L. In the first case it seems too good to be true, and I'm sure it will not last.
F. We can forget that.
L. Forget that.
F. But you should take pleasure in it—enjoy it while it's there.
L. Yes—but I don't. I suppose in a way I feel sort of insecure? You know, not quite sure.
F. What's likely to happen? What does insecure mean?
L. Well—I don't know exactly what insecure means in this context. Perhaps—I'll think about it—but one other thing which makes me feel uneasy is that I'm sort of afraid that my fluency won't last—that I'll slip back into—and stammer again.
F. I see.
L. If I'm talking fluently I feel that I haven't got real control over my fluency.

A very intriguing flat declaration of his view of himself as a core role stammerer. Also there is the recurrent suggestion that being fluent is wrong because it is pretending to be something he is not. Later in the same interview we get:

L. I am not really aware that it [speech] is getting better and better—if it wasn't for these ratings.
F. When you sit down and think about it . . .
L. When I sit down and think about it, or if, for example, I remember how I was, the last time I was here talking to you. I'm a jolly sight more fluent today probably than you can ever remember—yes, yes—and so I say to myself— 'well—this *must* be an improvement'—even although I want to think that it is

just a good patch. I must argue to myself that it's *not* a chance good patch and in fact it *is* improvement.

F. And it's a consistent thing—a gradual . . .

L. Improvement.

F. A gradual increase in fluency.

L. Yes, yes. But, you see, I can argue this intellectually and that's fair enough but to believe it is a different thing. Although I can argue intellectually that I am gradually improving—um—*I still feel a stammerer.*

Fluency is still very threatening and unacceptable. This leads him to show hostility in virtually denying the evidence that fluency is upon him. It is also threatening him because it is still less meaningful to him as a way of life than stuttering. As long as he still stutters or thinks himself a stutterer he can ward off the threat of imminent changes in his core role construing.

Session 11

Excerpts from this interview have to be limited because of the content of the discussion. But two of them show that there is an improvement both in the quality and in the complexity of construing. Luke is following through ideas about respect and so forth with more elaboration and is much more firm in the way he expresses himself, than in the earlier sessions.

Whereas in the last session he had nothing to contribute on the subject of the non-verbal aspects of fluency, such as hand gestures, tone of voice and so forth, he has clearly been thinking about this in the interval and volunteers the following.

L. I have found myself observing the way people handle conversation. Listening to the way the people I meet talk. But in particular on the radio. I find the conversation jolly interesting because people, say, when someone is being interviewed, the interviewer asks pertinent questions with seeming complete ease. I say to myself, I wouldn't know what to ask them! I found this situation very interesting, keeping the conversation going. And I've realize that it is probably a natural thing for people to do this at some stage of life. I'm not sure if they do it at one particular stage of their life or whether they do it all through their life, but it's probably a natural thing to imitate other people's conversations. Now, the interesting thing is that I think I am right in saying that, to the stammerer, the world of conversation doesn't exist. His world is the world of actions, isn't it? And I've always noticed that I have tended to imitate other people's actions and did think this is quite an interesting thing. Other people imitate other people by means of communicating by conversations, stammerers, or at least this particular one, tends to imitate other actions as a means of communication.

F. This whole art of conversation is something to be learned.

L. Yes, certainly. I feel at present that I'm still not getting sufficient fluency to be able to practice it, but I am storing up subconsciously little examples of the art of conversation to be used as soon as I am able.

F. I wish I had a camera. You are certainly using your hands a great deal more, especially that last bit. This is all part of the art of talking.

L. Actually, this is something I have been tending to concentrate on. But it does come naturally.

Session 13

He reports an unpleasant incident in a hotel while on holiday on the Continent, in which he was justifiably angry. He described how he 'saw the Manager and explained to him what had happened and generally complained and in a five minute conversation there was a hundred percent fluency'. I then asked how he explained this fluency:

F. Why should that incident have been so significant?

L. I think it probably illustrated to me that I could handle a fairly *aggressive* situation. Um it also probably reminded me that I could talk fluently.

*   *   *

F. I'm trying to think of the word you used before to deal with the aggressive situation. It's not primarily aggression, it's something to do with being master of the situation. I'm not quite sure what it was. Yes, it's a respect sort of thing. People are respected who stand up for their rights, who show they are not to be trifled with. This was an act of that nature, wasn't it? Highly important to show yourself that you can deal with such a situation from time to time.

The above was an attempt on my part to encourage him to relate the incident to something other than aggression. He normally fails to relate his way of speaking with the content of what he is saying or with the degree of conviction that he is right. I hoped that my offerings of other constructions within his repertoire would encourage him to elaborate on this theme.

L. I think this is shown by my wife who said she has known me for a year or more and never realized that there was an aggressive side to my personality.

F. Are you right in calling it aggression?

L. No, perhaps not, shall I say a *firmness*, a firm side to my personality. I think my wife thinks I'm a bit soft you know.

Session 15

The following long excerpt is given to show the considerable elaboration that has been taking place, perhaps started by the traumatic incident in the hotel. At first he tries to reach for a superordinate construct about stuttering (that it relates to somebody who wins sympathy by being inoffensive and frightened), and then generalizes this to voice production as a whole and imitates a "frightened voice". This indicates how superordinate his construing of stuttering is. He is attempting to relate it to a whole issue about personality, life style and to the purposes of social interaction. But the demonstration of a "frightened voice" is particularly interesting because it shows an increasing degree of freedom and a willingness to experiment in his personal presentation.

L. Last Tuesday evening I was thinking about my relationship towards other people and I made a brief note which I am frantically trying to decipher. Yes, that's it. It concerned, yes, that I usually find I am more fluent when I feel that I am the *master of the situation*. For example, if I was explaining some technical thing to you, I should probably explain it in pretty fluent language. For example again, an incident which occurred some time ago. When I was thinking about this, it sprang to mind that I could use it as an example. I've got my car parked in a place where there is a notice 'do not park here'. It is when I collect my wife in the evening. There are quite a lot of large lorries which park near where she works and it is where they want to park. One evening I went to park there and when the lorry driver wanted to get out, I just leaned out of the window and said 'shall I move my car back a bit so you can get out?' The point of this example is that there are two ways in which I can say 'shall I move my car?' There is (a) the way in which somebody would say it if they were afraid that they were in the wrong place, in an extremely frightened sort of way, or (b) the way in which a person would say it if they thought 'well it is all right for somebody to park here, it is not hurting anybody, but if you like I don't mind moving back a bit so that you can get out'. In the second case the person would be *master of the situation*. 'I don't mind moving back'—the other [imitates a frightened voice] 'I don't mind moving back'.

F. It's almost a matter of politeness really.

L. Yes it is, in the second case, in the first a matter of fear. So I think that probably basically in my character, in consistency with my character, I would have adopted the first and so I continue with this and say it is nice to be master of the situation and be a rather forceful character. I would have said that people who were forceful were not necessarily liked and I would have felt that people would be more inclined to like or feel sorry for the inoffensive little man who was frightened he was in the wrong place, rather than the chap who is a little more forceful and sure of himself. Now I believe that this is probably wrong. I believe that people probably respect a forceful person and certainly do not dislike them. Whereas the weak inoffensive little man is one who other people sort of despise rather than like. But I think it shows to a certain extent how my mind has worked in the past and certainly as far as stammering is concerned. The stammering man is rather like this weak inoffensive little man.

F. He can't be forceful can he.

L. Exactly. So I—what you can make of that little situation I do not know.

F. Well, what do you make of it?

L. Well, I think it is possibly a reason in the past that I have stammered, and possibly a reason why I wanted to be respected and this sort of thing. I think it all hinges on wanting to be liked and this sort of thing.

F. You said the reason why you stammered. I think you could equally well argue that the reason why you stammered was you tended to be rather diffident, because you couldn't put your point over concisely and so on.

L. I don't think that is true. Because when *I want to be angry and be forceful I can be perfectly fluent and be forceful*.

F. But you have to be angry.

L. Do I have to be angry? Yes, I probably do.

F. You couldn't be a firm person as a matter of course, you have to be worked up about something.

L. Yes, probably.

F. Do you think this represents some change?

L. I think that there has been a considerable change over my way of thinking about situations such as this. I have also got a much greater degree of insight into the way other people think.

F. Does your way of thinking influence your way of behaving?

L. I think probably not. Certainly I can say that the change in my way of thinking has not affected my fluency.

F. I was not particularly thinking of your fluency, but in that particular instance in the past you probably would have been the fearful one . . .

L. So it has changed me. It probably has. I was thinking more in terms of my general personality, whatever that is.

F. In this particular instance you were able to say 'shall I move' perfectly fluently.

L. It started off a—after I got the 'shall' out it was all right.

F. Sticking to this situation. Did it occur to you what sort of person this would be when you started to speak?

L. Yes it did.

F. Did you think there are two ways of doing this?

L. Yes I did.

F. What made you opt for the second?

L. Because I feel it's more in keeping with my character.

F. Is being forceful the same as being firm?

L. Yes, *I think* it is. When I mean being forceful, being firm, what I mean is being confident in oneself. Confident in one's—confident that one is doing the right thing or taking the right course of action.

F. And you think that appearing confident to other people too has the same effect. If you are confident in what you're doing, do you think other people will think you confident?

L. I think so.

F. If this is true, I think you said in the beginning that you thought your stammer related to when you were boss of the situation. Is this being boss of the situation this confidence and firmness?

He now goes on to elaborate at some length his construing of fluency and its relation to ideas of firmness, respect and so forth.

L. Yes, I think it is. Let's see now, let me just get my ideas straight. Yes, I think that what I mean is that when I feel *master of the situation* and am confident that whatever I say or do will be accepted and that people will continue to like me for what I say and do people will respect me. If I do not feel master of the situation I probably don't know quite how to put what I want to say and still be sure of retaining people's respect, sort of thing.

F. Are they not going to respect you because you can't put things properly? Or aren't you able to put things properly because you are not going to get their respect? Take—can you think of a situation in which you were not the master and were stammering.

L. No I can't I'm afraid, because all situations where this feeling of mastering the situation could have been in some doubt, I probably thought quite a lot about the situation beforehand and decided on a way of approach whereby I could be master of the situation. I may have subsequently lost the mastery because I stammered but, to me, because I stammered, these situations are recalled as being situations in which I stammered through habit or something like this. It's a little complex isn't it?

F. Yes, I'm not too clear. We have got a situation in which you say to yourself 'I'm not going to be the master of the situation'.

L. No—oh dear me, I don't know really.

F. Can we take the example of the car. You worked out that you were going to be the master of the situation. Supposing you had decided 'no', how would the situation have been different?

L. I imagine I would have stammered very much indeed. I imagine that self consciously it would have been something like this. 'Am I going to be master of the situation? No I am not. Therefore I am not going to get the person's respect. If I don't get his respect then I may as well get his sympathy and stammer.'

F. What we have got to find out is what determines this monitoring—what made you decide 'yes, I am going to be master of this situation'.

L. I think it must be to a certain extent—well knowledge of another person's reactions, knowledge of others' reactions to me as master of the situation and not master of the situation. He will probably respect me for being master of the situation but not if I were not. And so, also, I said, in fact, was I doing any real harm in parking my car or not. I mean to say, if one took it back to one's child-hood would someone say 'oh you naughty boy for parking your car there'.

F. Probably yes. If you take the police to be the adult. But what is the important thing surely is that adults do not work as children work. You can look at a situation and say 'well I'm not supposed to be here, but I'm calling for my wife and I've got to park somewhere and I'm not doing any harm and I'm willing to move away'. It's perfectly reasonable.

Here is a clear example of how Luke now accepts the idea that his construing of the construction processes of another determines whether he stammers or not. He then elaborates on a second causative factor— whether he is in the right or not.

L. Yes, I said there's no reasonable reason why I should not park here and so I'm master of the situation. If there had been a good reason why I should not park there, then I should probably feel I was not master of the situation. Because somebody could come along and say 'look you're definitely wrong here'.

F. Yes, what is at the back of my mind is that one can be master of any situation you want. So what the child does, and possibly the stammerer to some extent, is to impose right and wrong on a situation. This then determines whether you are master of the situation or not. But if you do what you did and stop using right and wrong—('you're wrong to park there because it says no parking, but adults ignore that sort of thing') and work out whether it is *reasonable* to park there or not, all's well.

L. Actually, I think that I can probably soon turn a situation in which I was not master into a situation in which I was master again. I think the problem must lie then in situations which I do not know whether I am going to be master or not. I, so probably—oh I don't know. If I had three situations then say, one situation when one is certain one is going to be master, for example, if I were asked to give a talk on a subject near and dear to my heart; the situation where one is not master—in which case I would be very able to turn it into one where I was master—I think so anyway, and then in that case one must have an intermediate situation in which one doesn't know if one is going to be master or not. So what is the significance of this situation compared with the others.

F. I can think of one in which you are equals, there isn't going to be a master.

L. Ohhhh. Yes. Yes. I think that this is beginning to clarify. Certainly in the two extreme cases I was thinking about, master of the situation and situations which I could easily turn myself into master, are exactly the same because in both I end up by being master. Then there is the situation in which the other person is going to be master of the situation and remain the master of the situation.

F. But you can't think of an example.

L. No. And there is also the situation where we are equals.

F. What happens in that situation.

L. [pause] I rather imagine that this is the situation which I would not be particularly happy with.

F. Can you think of an example?

L. [pause] No I can't really. But what bothers [extreme stammer] goodness me— is that in this, there is the underlying indication that one person must be master and the other not and this is not necessarily so is it.

F. No, I was not going to bring it up. I mean it is not what most people would take into account, but I can quite understand how most stammerers have learned to take it into account and why it becomes very important. They are so insecure about anything to do with communication. The minute you start getting anything approaching fluency you realize that it is not important. You start to act to the best of your ability in that situation. You weigh it up, decide what is best, and so on. Not saying 'now then I am going to be master of the situation'.

L. Yes. Something else which has just come into my mind. As regards parking a car is concerned, it is a situation which one can weigh up upon concrete evidence. But there are situations which involve just speech, that is to say a verbal battle or indeed a verbal exchange not necessarily a battle. Again one feels one wants to be master of the situation or at least master of the impression one conveys in conversation, but of course for the stammerer this is not very easy.

F. No. But you see just as with the driver, apart from the very beginning you were fluent. I say you were fluent because you had decided that it was OK, you were not doing any harm, not that you were confident because you were fluent. In the same way, in conversation, if you sum up the person in that situation as one with whom you can give as good as you get, then you will be fluent. If you decide 'oh dear, I am not sure now, this man has a reputation for this that and the other . . .' I would predict that you would stammer badly.

L. It probably is so and of course one has the situation where one cannot sum this up beforehand.

F. And this may be the situation in which you do not know, which will be a tricky one, particularly if you insist on summing it up in terms of who is going to be master.

L. Or actually not in terms of who is going to be boss but in terms of 'at the end of this situation will this person still like me'. Certainly, I think that I would feel a bit upset or a bit uncomfortable if I thought somebody went away absolutely hating me.

F. But what I think will happen and what has happened a great deal already—a little while ago everybody had to respect you, had to be *seen* to respect you, now this is no longer true. There are many situations in which this is irrelevant, they respect you if you show yourself to be competent and so on. So what is happening is a narrowing down. But there is still the group in the middle who you can't decide about. But I'm quite confident that as this is whittled down more and more so these will disappear too. Do you know what I mean?

L. I do indeed.

F. To begin with respect was such an all embracing thing, everything was seen in terms of respect, now it is less important but it hasn't been eliminated.

L. I can think of a good example of this. When I first started seeing you I felt that whenever I went into a restaurant that I would have liked special treatment, a red carpet swished out in front of me and so forth, but now I just don't think about it. As far as the waiters are concerned I am just one of a number of people, give my order and that's all.

He has clearly come a long way from the man who wanted respect at any price but inconsistencies keep showing through in his construing system.

In the following extract he first of all gives the argument that he falls back on his stutter to cover up his inadequacy—so the stutter *disguises* his inadequacy. But then he goes on to say that if somebody met him as a fluent person, they would accept him *for what he is* and the idea of an inferiority complex would be absolute rubbish. However, if they met him as a stammerer, this would not necessarily be true. In short, stuttering is now being looked on not as a disguise of inadequacy or inferiority, but as an index or revelation of inadequacy in its own right. This seems to suggest that he is exploring two alternative lines of implication but hasn't yet elaborated one successfully and thereby been able to discover the other. If stuttering helps him out in situations in which he finds construing difficult then he would have to accept the implication that as he elaborates his construing system, his stuttering will become unnecessary. If stuttering is the result of inadequacy, then he has the problem of defining what that inadequacy is. In some theoretical frameworks this type of construing would be given as an example of the "neurotic paradox". This is our recognition that the person is legitimately balanced between two interpretations of his life situation. What seems to become clear from this is that it is the interpretation of the behaviour that keeps it going, not the presence or absence of some reinforcement as such.

L. Sometime ago I came and my speech was pretty poor and I put it down to the fact that I had just visited my parents in the West Country and I was back having had a long hard drive and I was feeling tired. I think at the time you said you did predict that after a few days of rest from the drive it would improve and I thought it would. But, in fact, my speech didn't. Well, this sort of feeling of tiredness I think it may be, in fact, just a general feeling of lack of confidence. Oh, yes, it all comes flooding back. I must catch it before it goes again. Yes. If I feel inadequate to cope with situations, say, this general tired feeling—inadequacy—no mastery—then I would fall back to being a—fall back to my stammer to cover up for my inadequacy—that's it, yes.

F. An excuse, or something—sympathy aroused . . .

L. Yes, I'd say if a situation arises whereby I'm to exert my rights or any situation at all in which if I've got this general feeling of lack of confidence or lack of forcefulness even something like this, then I'd revert back to this 'I can't be bothered' —something like that—feeling generally tired out. If I stammer, everything's all right—you know.

F. It's easier.

L. Easier, yes. Exactly. It is, in fact, easier for me to stammer than for me to arouse myself from this general lethargic lack of confidence state.

*   *   *

L. I think that if somebody met me as a fluent person, they would accept me for what I am, and the whole idea of inferiority complex would be absolute rubbish. If they met me as a stammerer [sigh], I don't think it would necessarily be true.

At the end of this interview there was an interchange between Luke and myself which has been likened to a session of rational–emotive psychotherapy. He attempts to relate certain constructions about merit to very concrete elements. He tries hard to identify a very complex role with very simple pieces of evidence such as how old one is or how one dresses. It is like saying that all there is to being a soldier is wearing a uniform.

L. Yes, I think this is quite an important factor as far as I'm concerned—are people still seeing me as being immature, or as a youngster—a young adolescent, or something like this. Are people still going to say 'Oh—he's only a youngster' [laughs].

F. But they can't if you're a scientist.

L. No—they can't—and so when I tell them that I'm a scientist they think 'but he's only a youngster—he can't be a scientist—he's only a laboratory assistant really'.

F. [laughter] But then they say 'but he doesn't talk like a lab. assistant'. [laughter] —so what are they going to end up with?

L. I suppose that I could probably arrive at a conclusion—say 'Oh, he's a lab. assistant' and after that disregard everything else which said differently. Perhaps I imagined other people would do this.

F. But you just now said that maybe you'd always thought of yourself as twenty-one or something—you hadn't really thought about it before. But why should other people think this? You don't look twenty-one.

L. Because—but—I don't think that I look twenty-one.

F. Why should they think it—I'm puzzled.

L. I said this because I had not sufficiently thought about the situation myself. What I said was in fact the old original ideas which have in the past five minutes replaced . . .

F. Yes—I'm pushing it in front of you again. I repeat my question—why should people think you are . . .

L. What?

F. Twenty-one. You've just brought up the argument—'Ah, yes—he says he's a scientist but after all he can't be—he's so young he must be a lab. assistant'.

L. Well actually again I'm side-tracking—I didn't put a specific date of twenty-one or an age of twenty-one.

F. How high do you go?

L. I put 'he is too young'.

F. But why—with most of your arguments there's some evidence to support them—why should you be thought too young to be a scientist? Are scientists all so old? They're not to me—any more than doctors are.

L. Because you see I've not been prepared to accept that people accept me in as grand a role as a scientist, perhaps they see me as being too young.

F. And I say—why on earth should they see you as being too young? I mean, if you put up excuses, you must allow your excuses to be attacked.

L. Sure—yes.

F. And, you've got to defend them—why should they see . . .

L. Well [laugh] [long silence] there's no reason why they should. It's just that it is one possible excuse for people not seeing me in as grand a role.

F. What comes to me—you know what comes to me?

L. No.

F. That it's not people who don't see you in a grand role—it's you . . .

L. Oh yes, yes.

F. And this is the reason why we've got to search for all these excuses—which are quite invalid excuses, and *obviously* invalid excuses.

L. This is true.

F. Now—the implications of you accepting 'you' in this grand role are what? What is a scientist in your view?

L. [sigh] I don't quite—see what you're getting at.

F. Right—you used the words 'see me in such a grand role as a scientist', or you used the words 'grand role'.

L. Yes, yes.

F. All right—we'll accept this—it is a high position in society. Why is it difficult for you to see yourself in it? Why is it difficult for you to accept that you are in this role? And therefore to get at the reasons we can ask how do I see other scientists.

L. Yes. The reason, I think, why I don't see myself in this role is because I'd like to be—I'd like to occupy a high position in society, and I'd like to believe that I did. But I'd rather not believe it in case it turned out to be untrue and all my hopes were dashed to the ground. You know what I mean? It's something—the Bible says—when you go to a wedding feast and you don't go right up to the very front in case somebody says 'Would you move back a bit—there are some more important people' and you sit right at the very back so that the usher can say 'you're more important now—would you move up a bit'. It's this sort of thing—playing safe or something—so you understand what I mean?

This seems to relate to his construing of being genuine—not only must one not pretend to be something one is not, but one must not make a mistake about what one is.

F. I understand what you mean but I don't think we've got it absolutely clear.

You see you *are* a scientist. This is not a disputed fact at all. Therefore, what—I'm not too sure about it—what the dispute is about.

L. OK then—the dispute is about the position in society which I hold and which other people see me as holding.

F. As a scientist—this is what we're discussing.

L. Yes, OK—all right—but in my reply to you I was taking the argument a stage further—OK, a scientist has a certain position in society and that's fixed and that's fair enough. There's nothing you can do about it. It's laid down. There is a law which says a scientist has this position and that's fair enough. The thing is that what I'm concerned about is the position of a person in society and that's this person—myself.

F. Yes, I say you are a scientist.

L. But I will then say a scientist isn't the only factor which determines a person's position in society. It's not the only factor. There are factors such as personal appearance.

F. You can't have it that way—why have it both ways. [laughter] If it is laid down by law that a scientist occupies this position in society as opposed to that position or that position, then you cannot go and say—'Ah but there's more to it than being a scientist—it depends on . . .'

L. OK. OK. A scientist occupies this position in society provided that he is well-dressed, and passable in comparison with other members of the public who also hold that same level in society.

F. I think what you've got to do now is to work out a character sketch of a scientist. What is a scientist?

L. I don't think it is this at all—a scientist is a chap who's got one particular type of job like a doctor or an accountant, or something like that. His job . . .

F. No—you gave me 'the grand role in society'—your very words.

L. [silence] You see, what I'm trying to do is put a condition on it. And having put these lists of conditions I then have to check myself to see if I satisfy all these conditions and probably some of these conditions I'm not sure if I satisfy them or not. And therefore I have to pretend to myself that perhaps I don't satisfy them—then I'll say to myself 'far better for me to say that I *don't* satisfy them and perhaps sometime in the future I may be proved wrong than to say that I do satisfy them and then to be proved that I don't satisfy them! This is what I'm trying to do.

F. Yes—but being a scientist is a bit of paper—A, B, C, D, E, F, all that incorporates being a scientist—so you say 'Well I've got a bit of paper—what about A, B, C, D, E, F'?

L. It isn't quite like that, I don't think. The important thing here is a level of social status.

F. A grand role?

L. Yes—a grand role which means it's got a high level of social status . . .

F. This is not the problem—it's there.

L. These two descriptions—a 'a grand role' and 'high social status' are the same.

F. Do you live up to them? Is that the sort of question?

L. [Laughter]

F. Are you worthy of it?

L. I'm certainly worthy of being a scientist, yes. The thing is am I worthy of . . .

F. —occupying that . . .

L. Occupying that role which could be . . .

F. which goes with being a scientist . . .

L. which could go with being a scientist—provided . . .
F. —it isn't automatic . . .
L. —you are well-dressed and that sort of thing.

This is an extension of the theme of a previous interview in which how he was dressed determined the likelihood of people being aggressive toward him—and his inability to know what to do in response to it. Similarly with pretence—people may say 'who does he think he is, pretending to be something he is not?'

F. So we are back. What I want you to do during the week is to put down all the characteristics that enable a person to be worthy of occupying that grand role in society—as they occur to you—put them down.
L. Yes—right—I'd better get my ideas clear on this before I put things down. Yes [writing]. Yes. So what I've put down is 'A scientist could occupy a grand role in society on the following conditions', and then, 'what are these conditions?' Yes. And of course the conditions can be summarized in that he should behave in all ways the same as other members of society occupying the same role but who are not necessarily scientists.
F. Yes. Being a scientist makes it potentially possible for you to occupy that grand role in society if as well as being a scientist you are also intelligent, dum dum dum.
L. Yes.
F. So we're back to status.
L. Back to status again.
F. It seems to me quite clear now that on many things you are much happier and more confident.
L. Yes. I am. I don't know about this idea of status. It's—there are things I'd like to do which I am financially unable to do. That is to say—in this grand role in society one would automatically be rich.
F. All scientists are not rich.
L. They are not—no . . .
F. I mean—isn't it going back to childhood—aren't you trying to occupy the squire's role and feeling uncomfortable about it?
L. Yes.
F. "Wealth", it you think about it, is not a prerequisite—desirable—but not a prerequisite for occupying that role.
L. Yes,—desirable, but not—yes.

A great deal of what Luke has been saying could be construed as simple snobbery. But to do so would be an error. The snobbery is not simple, it is a very complicated system with, as yet relatively unexplored, ties with values about himself and about his own identity.

Session 16

Luke in this session is implying that not to stammer is to feel confident, or at least not to feel a *lack of* confidence. This suggests that there still is a massive unawareness of mood, posture, experience and feeling as related to the actual content, quality and nature of what is going on between people and therefore that lacking in confidence is just as frequently a problem for the nonstammerer as for the stammerer. This seems to be part of this very oversimplified *master of the situation* versus *not master of the situation* construction, which is still, as yet, very poorly elaborated

L. I feel sure that whenever I do come to speak fluently I will feel, shall we say, confident. Whenever I have something to say I'll feel completely confident.

F. In yourself or that your speech will be all right?

L. In myself.

F. Why should that be? You'll be just a normal human being—they're not confident all the time are they?

L. No. Well in that case, I would not *lack confidence* shall we say.

F. Yes. I can see that. What you mean is that if it's an over-riding characteristic you will be confident in all situations?

L. No. But it does mean that I will not feel the lack of confidence that I feel now— this type of thing.

Session 17

Luke is now becoming more and more open and definite about his search for status and the enormous importance it has for him. This means that he is recognizing the superordinate quality of how other people see him, or how he thinks they see him. The difficulty still is that he has no constructions of other people through which he can "filter" their opinions of him and make sense of them and use their reactions as evidence. In a curious way, he seems to have to accept at face value what he thinks other people might think of him, because he can't relate it to what he thinks *they* are. He is still as much at sea in relation to the Sociality Corollary as he was at the beginning.

However, the following excerpt shows that he is now seriously contemplating the possibility of being a fluent speaker. He is contemplating issues like whether his speech will be refined, whether he will be a chatterbox and whether he will then be able to accept that he is a person who merits being in a position of authority, and so on. In previous interviews he safeguarded himself by coming down in the last analysis with the view that he was, and might well remain, a stammerer. But here the vision of himself as a fluent speaker seems to be looming up. At this point Bannister predicted that there would be so much threat in this situation (as defined by Kelly) that it would cause a relapse. He was right.

F. So you are beginning to enter the shoes of this other person?

L. Yeah. I think so.

F. I wondered because last week, when I asked you, you were quite sure that you were very much still a stammerer.

L. Yes—I know. I think that I can now imagine what it will be like to be fluent, and I also feel that there is a very high probability I *will* become fluent. This, I think is a quite interesting thing, because I think if you look back through your notes you will see that about three or so weeks ago you asked me if I could imagine what it would be like to be fluent. And I said that I wouldn't *like* to imagine it because I was not confident that I would ever become fluent. But now I am pretty well confident.

F. Yes—there was a time, wasn't there, when your fluency, or patches of fluency, were rather alarming to you. You were very uneasy about them. They felt unnatural.

L. Yes. Yes. Yes. Yes. I think the thing is that we have now got the cause of my stammer down to such a fine degree that we're able to practically pinpoint the causes of my stammering in various situations. And—er—that's a good thing as far as I am concerned. It has given me confidence.

I asked about how his wife viewed the prospect of a fluent husband.

F. I expect she is looking forward to this day.

L. I think so—yes. In fact I'm absolutely certain that she'll have such a chatter-box on her hands that she won't get a word in edgeways. [laughter]

F. You may go through a chatterbox phase, but it won't last unless you're basic-ally a chatterbox. I don't think you probably are.

L. Perhaps not, I don't know.

F. What about other aspects of your fluent speech?

L. Well, it will be refined. What I mean is not coarse or vulgar—the accent will not be coarse or vulgar. It will indicate some force of character. That is to say, the kind of person who is in a position of authority—and is probably aware of the fact—also accepts it—and does not think that other people will think him *big-headed*.

Session 18

The predicted relapse occurred. Having last time taken a very positive step toward construing himself as a fluent speaker, he now takes one step backwards. He becomes concerned with situations in which he is listening to fluent speakers and contrasting himself with them. The description of listening to the man asking for the reference over the telephone is the first time he has talked of the way somebody else speaks. It is as if, now that he is faced with being at the contrast pole (the fluent speaker pole) he is forced to look at elements at this end and compare them with him-self. He finds that the contrast, which after all is the essence of the construct itself, is still there between him and fluent people.

L. Last Tuesday we asked the question 'why am I not a fluent speaker?' The asking of this question has had quite a startling effect on me—the stammer's got worse.

F. Can you explain it?

L. Well—many situations occurred in which I heard other people talking or I imagined myself in situations where I would have to have a conversation. These situations I feel very unhappy about. I feel very uneasy about them.

F. Can you give me an example?

L. Well, yes. The one I took particular note of was an example of where somebody else was holding a conversation which I could not have done. This chap at work had a reference which he wanted to check. He phoned the technical library and said to them 'Oh, I've got a reference I'd like you to check for me please—it's author so and so and it's called so and so—could you look it up and give me the exact reference'. And I thought to myself then—you know—'I couldn't have done that'.

He then goes on to give other examples of the contrast between himself and others and how he could not do the things they do. It appears that he is aware of the threat implicit in the situation for him. I follow this up with an attempt to reduce the threat, by giving him the Kellian explanation.

L. I think I may stammer more because I—I don't know—I've probably been I probably haven't had the fact that one day I would be a fluent speaker brought home to me with a bang—you know what I mean? And—er—I suddenly sort of began to say 'Ah yes,—I'm going to be a fluent speaker'.

F. Help!!

L. Yes [Laughs]

According to the present theory of stuttering, the confrontation with the other 'fluent self' has brought about the sudden realization or *awareness of an imminent comprehensive reduction of the total number of predictive implication of the personal construct system* (Hinkle, 1965). In this therapeutic approach, one of the main problems is how to avoid pushing the person along too fast. He must have established *sufficient* implications of being a symptom-free person to be able to face the prospect without being threatened. Threat is seen as making the person retreat into the self he knows.

Session 19

The attempt to reduce the threatening nature of fluency appeared to work, or something did, as his speech improved during the week. One repeated theme in many previous interviews comes out again clearly in this one. Luke tries to work out the implications of *status* in a very concretistic way. He wants operational definitions, subordinate constructions of *status* and being *worthy of respect* which are indisputable. These include one's profession, dress, class and so forth. He can then, he thinks, be quite certain of being able to predict the other person's reactions to himself. However, he eventually comes specifically to the problem which is that 'I can't predict what these—or at least I can't predict what people's reactions will be to me in *every* situation'. This is an admission of the inadequacy of the kind of subordinate implications for which he has been trying to get validation.

L. What one wants is to be happy that he's respected all the time and that—yes— happy that he's respected all the time. He knows how people are going to react to what he says and does so that he need never do anything which people would react to in the wrong way.

F. That's utopia, isn't it?

L. Yes [uncertainly]. I think that everybody—I think everybody has got their own particular scapegoats so that probably everybody has got their group of people to whom they do not care what they say. They've also got a group of people to whom they are careful about what they say or how they behave so that the reaction is always favourable.

F. As favourable as possible.

L. As favourable as possible.

F. They can't guarantee it, can they?

L. No [uncertainly]. What am I trying to say—I think that I'm slowly trying to get around to saying that perhaps the situation is that I can't predict what these—or at least I can't predict what people's reaction will be to me in every situation.

F. Nor can anyone.

L. Probably I feel that I am less—well—I think that I feel—what am I trying to say—that I would not be happy that I know—I'm not happy that I can predict the behaviour of other people towards me with as great an accuracy—or with as great confidence as other people.

Session 20

In this session he again changes from the construct *wins respect* or *has status* to *create a favourable impression* versus *creates an unfavourable impression*. This does not seem like merely a piece of relabelling. It looks as if he is trying to get a more permeable, looser construction which will give him more room to manoeuvre than the old construction *respect*. For example, when he is trying to think up instances which might create an unfavourable impression he stresses that he doesn't have to be concerned about "the finer points of etiquette". By particularly specifying situations likely to result in an unfavourable impression he seems to be trying to make the construct lopsided. He is saying that most things create a favourable impression and only a few very rare and special things create the unfavourable impression. Therefore, the whole social situation is not so risky as he used to think it was because most behaviours will work all right in creating the favourable impression.

Session 21

His speech improved to a new level during the previous week and in this session he introduces the idea that he may be resisting cure. Only now can it be discussed openly. This is because it would have been completely unacceptable to him as an idea if he were confronted with it before having had a chance to explore and experiment with ideas about stuttering and fluency and, in fact, elaborate the idea for himself.

L. Now those situations in which I am most likely to stutter. The first is when I tell a lie, which ties up with leading people up the garden path—*pretending*. But this is not telling direct lies. And certainly the idea of fraud is tied in with this again—to bluff my way out of a situation. Now, this sort of thing will tie in probably with the reason for my bad speech to you when I first come in—I have a confession to make—off we go. I sort of feel that in the past I probably should have taken a more active interest in trying to get rid of my stammer than I have. I don't know whether this is true or not but I feel that I should have been, or at least certainly been—no—I feel that I'm capable to thinking about the situation during the week and trying to work out some new ideas—and in general help you along as much as possible—and I've been a bit on the lazy side about this in the past. So over Christmas I thought 'enough of this laziness' and my wife got on to me as well and said I was lazy. I sort of jot things down, but the point is that previously I've sort of come in sort of wondering 'is she thinking that I'm a little bit on the lazy side and not doing anything'? So in a way I've been trying to bluff around the fact that I've not been terrifically active.

F. But as you've sat here—you have tried hard—so then it was all right? Why laziness? People aren't lazy for no reason are they? Why do you think you didn't think harder about things?

L. I don't know whether I agree with you on that 'people aren't lazy for no reason'.

F. You came wanting to get rid of your stammer—it wasn't thrust upon you like a boy at school—to do his homework or something.

L. No, no.

F. You took an active step.

L. Yes. It could well be in fact, that this is not so much lack of interest, but certainly lack of wanting to get down and do something—do you know what I mean? I could quite easily say to myself driving home from work 'right, tonight I'm going to sit down and sort out my stammer'. But when it came to the time, then I didn't feel like it and I think that this could well be the fact that probably somewhere, subconsciously, I didn't want to get rid of it because it was—you know—just this sort of thing. That there was something in the fluent world that I was afraid of.

Towards the end of the interview he introduces, also for the first time, the construct *human*. This represents an elaboration well beyond the original construction of wanting people to like him. It is as if he also wants to like *them*. Additionally, it contains the idea of certain kinds of relationship as having value in themselves quite apart from their utility in getting things done and so forth. It is almost as if he is toying with the idea of a non-manipulative relationship. And if stammering is viewed as a form of manipulation by the stammerer, this could be very important.

This excerpt comes after he had been making some notes.

L. So at the end of this I conclude: Surely the whole basis of this is not knowing the other person's reaction to what I'm going to say. And this ties in with making—with knowing the nicest way to ask people—to get them to do what I want to do—either having the correct approach by saying exactly what you want—or having what I call the *human* approach. And that's it.

F. Did you say "human"?

L. Yes—that's it—I thought—just as I was going to say 'human' I thought 'that's a funny word to have used'.

F. Why the word 'funny'.

L. Because 'human' means—would be tied up with humanity and asking somebody to do something in a nice way isn't necessarily tied up with humanity—is it? So why—.

F. But you wouldn't have written it if you hadn't meant it.

L. I wouldn't have written it—

F. What does it mean?

L. I suppose it is 'human'—yes, it probably was what I meant actually when I think about it. A human approach—it's the right word. It's in a way a philanthropic approach—that's a bad word as well. But certainly being nice to people.

Session 22

This session included the elicitation and laddering of constructs for the third NS-grid.

Having played about in the previous interview with '*human*' as a way of trying to deal with his great concern about what other people will think of him, he now experiments with an alternative idea. This is simply not caring what other people think about him. It is also clear that the implications of this look rather strange and worrisome to him. This new construction arose during the elicitation of constructs for the NS-grid.

F. These two are *physically strong* and this one is *physically weak*.

L. Physically *not strong* rather.

F. Right. These next ones now.

L. Could I just go back here again and sort out this physically strong thing again. It's not physical strength I think—I'm afraid that I'm a bit confused here—I see something between myself and this one and a weakness between myself and this one and a weakness between myself and this one. But I can't determine what it is.

F. Well, shall we leave it for the moment and come back to it? So here are three more.

L. So this one—yes. These two have the weakness associated with this one.

F. Physical weakness.

L. Yes physical weakness.

F. Can you not see more clearly what it is?

L. I wonder if it is carefreeness [a very bad stammer indeed]

F. That didn't sound very carefree [laughter]

L. No, that was the worst stammer for ages. It is absolutely amazing, because I cannot understand why carefreeness should be so significant, especially when I think it is a good thing to be carefree and in fact I did identify myself with the carefree person.

F. So where are we now?

L. *Physically strong* should be *carefree*.

F. Versus?

L. I don't know—sober, or even—what is it—sort of—the type of thing that has all the care's of the world on its shoulders—yes, *sober*.

(another triad offered)

L. Again this *carefree-sober* one.
F. Nothing else?
L. Nothing else. I can't understand why my subconscious should latch on to care-free in such a significant way.
(the laddering then goes ahead)
F. Which would you prefer to be a *strong-sure* person or a *weak-unsure* person?
L. The strong.
F. Right—why?
L. [long silence]. I think it's basically because then I wouldn't care what other people thought of me.
F. Why is it preferable not to care—than to care what other people think of you?
L. [silence] Because it would save me a lot of mental effort. The person who doesn't care what other people think about him just goes and does whatever he wants to—is able to indulge in himself or—indulge as much as he likes without giving a thought to the consequences which is—although for the sake of society it's not a good thing—as far as the individual's concerned it's prob-ably a—it's certainly far easier than—than—I was going to say—having to take other people into account. But more what I mean is, taking notice of other people's criticisms.

Session 24

Elicitation and laddering of constructs for the third S-grid take place during this session. After previous rather disastrous flirtation with the vision of fluency, Luke comes face to face with it again.

L. Last night I had an experience of perfect fluency—I didn't realize it was a "I" until a long time afterwards. And I was thinking 'crikey—I didn't think about stammering at all'. I often have situations where I will be fluent but I'm always conscious of the fact that I do stammer and that at any time I may start to stammer.

(Note: he did not rate his best for the week as I)

> The situation, to be exact, was this. My wife and I were out in the car trying to find a house to visit somebody—we hadn't been there before—we'd been given the number and the address—and some instructions. I misunderstood the instructions and we were hareing about trying to look for it, and it was in fact over here—sort of thing. We eventually got to a post-office. My wife went in to ask where it was while I sat in the car . . . I could see the chap who was in there was giving her a lot of directions from the map and I thought 'Oh dear' [laughter] 'we're not going to be much better off!' So I went in and the chap showed me the map and showed me where it was and I could see where I had gone wrong and so ensued a conversation lasting about three minutes in which he explained the best way for me to get there and I said 'I know such and such a road'—that sort of thing and I also had a laugh and explained where I had gone wrong because the road I used to know sort of did that and—but they'd built a new by-pass around it and I went down it and did all sorts of odd things. But this was a conversation in which I suppose my total speaking time added together would have been at least in the order of one and a half minutes— which is fair old time really—and it was completely fluent—and also I didn't think about stammering at all.

F. Did your wife confirm that it was completely fluent?

L. She didn't say it was completely fluent in so many words, but afterwards when I thought about it I said 'My speech in that shop was quite good—wasn't it?' and she said 'Yes—it was' so I don't know whether it was completely fluent or not, but I am . . .

F. Except that you're so often completely, or nearly fluent with her aren't you?

L. Yes.

F. So she wouldn't be surprised—she wouldn't know the difference, in you. You weren't paying attention to it this time whereas before you'd paid attention to it.

L. She might not have noticed—quite. But I'm absolutely convinced that I was one hundred per cent fluent.

F. Is this the first time it's happened? That you're aware it's happened?

L. Yes—certainly.

F. That's a good step.

L. It is happening to a certain extent now—actually—that sort of thing.

F. Once you've made this step you realize it's very important.

L. Yes—but I also think I can tell the reason why as well. It goes back to this sort of thing about whether *I like to be liked*, and this in fact—*not caring what other people think of you*—this sort of thing.

It would seem that here he was really able to experiment with the construction of *not caring* which he was able to put into words at the last session.

L. At that time we'd been driving around in the rush hour traffic and I wanted to find this place—and I was a bit fed up and I didn't really care what anybody thought of me anyway. And so this was certainly the reason why I had this fluency because my mental state was this somewhat—well certainly I didn't care what anybody thought of me. An interesting thing here is this, that whilst I don't know why—but I got the impression that this chap's wife—who was also serving behind the counter or something *was looking at me as though I was a little bit odd*. Now what I was doing I don't know. Also I got the impression that the chap was looking at me in rather an odd way. Now normally this would have bothered me, but at that time it didn't bother me at all—I thought 'if they want to look at me in an odd way—they can'. I meant to ask my wife if, in fact I was talking extra loud or if there was anything odd about the way I behaved, but unfortunately I forgot to ask her.

F. Do you really think they were looking at you oddly or was it that the situation was an odd one *to you*. Here, for the first time you were being fluent, you were aware of something unusual and you put it onto the people, do you really think that they were looking at you oddly?

L. That's very interesting. I don't know. I see what you mean. You see, normally, if I want to be liked—this sort of thing—even if I appear to be talking fluently I'll probably say odd little things or adopt certain attitudes or something so that people will like me, and people will be responsive to this. People will, say, smile at me if I smile at them—something like that. But of course in this situation last night I didn't bother with this sort of thing. So, therefore I— yes—that's perfectly true isn't it—so therefore I wouldn't expect my normal, liking, smiling reactions sort of thing.

F. For the first time you have have been getting a normal reaction to an ordinary person who has come to ask the way—which is unusual for you.

L. My wife does say that sometimes I do talk a bit loud and I wondered if in fact I was shouting my head off in the shop.

F. I doubt if you were shouting your head off and I doubt if people would look oddly if someone talks a bit loudly—this is something that you can come to terms with when you're confident about speaking. You can modulate your voice according to how you want it. I doubt if you were. I think your wife would have said 'Yes, it was fine but you were shouting a bit'.

L. Yes—I don't know really—perhaps not—not necessarily so.

F. You might have been shouting but I don't think they would have looked at you oddly—they might have thought you were deaf perhaps—and people who are deaf shout a bit.

L. Yes.

F. But you don't look at *them* oddly. I think it's quite interesting that you may have been getting ordinary, common or garden looks, which you're not used to. In fact, very unused to. Because, on the whole, people *don't* react to others and this is something stammerers don't understand—normally speaking you get fairly expressionless faces.

L. [silence]

F. Unless you go out of your way to establish a relationship. It's worth thinking about. 'Oddly'. Maybe they weren't looking oddly—maybe they were looking naturally.

L. Quite—it's *fantastic*.

This was considered to be a very important episode. Luke tried hard to make it out to be atypical in the realm of fluency by talking of "odd" reactions. He was offered the alternate construction that the reactions to him were not "odd" but, in fact, what he may expect from others in similar situations when he talks as others do. Maybe he was shouting, or being too "firm", but this did not matter. These things could be dealt with later. As these episodes were so rare, it was felt important that he elaborate his construing of *others* to his fluency and not concentrate on his construing of himself. Having tried to suggest he construe the reactions to him as something he may expect another time, we return to discussing how *he* felt.

F. Did this fluency give you a comfortable sort of feeling?

L. Oh yes. Quite comfortable. I think I said some things I probably shouldn't have said, in-so-much as the chap—you know—had a great climb to get out this map and it was all falling to pieces and had to be pieced together again and I said 'tatty old map—isn't it?' Of course I shouldn't have criticized his map because after all his map was going to save us time. I thought afterwards I shouldn't have said that.

F. But again it's interesting because you've got to learn these things. When fluency comes I always want to put muzzles on people because they're so pleased about being able to speak that they don't think about what they're going to say.

You know, as in this sort of situation—and I think you're at that border-line now and you have to think not 'can I say it properly' but 'what am I going to say'.

L. Yes—I don't think that this one situation has given me sufficient confidence.

He is not yet ready to buy fluency lock stock and barrel.

F. No—but I'm saying there will be more.

L. Yes. Provided I am in the same state of mind as I was then.

F. Oh yes. But states of mind are funny things. They're funny things in that as you've experienced this once it will tend to come back again. The difficulty is getting in that frame of mind in the first instance when it hasn't been experienced before.

L. Yes.

Session 25

The main points in this interview were the use, for the first time, of the role construct of 'diplomat' and that he had another experience of fluency.

Session 26

The previous experiences of fluency may have resulted in a nightmare he had.

L. I had a nightmare of unusual intensity, reminiscent of those suffered in child-hood. . . . I can see myself standing in our sitting-room screaming and stamping and jumping up and down with rage and my parents and the two evacuees sort of looking at me and sort of laughing.

In construct theory terms, this experience can be seen as Luke's reaction to having had a glimpse of significant chaos ahead of him. This may have resulted from a steady build up of evidence that he might actually become a fluent speaker and this was still a pretty meaningless life for him to lead or it may have been because of something said in the previous interview when he was given an example of a stammerer who virtually became fluent overnight when he reconstrued his father as an equal rather than as a superior. However, there is no direct evidence that this was the cause.

One point to be noted is that the significance of the nightmare was not explored although Luke wanted to dwell on it. It was deliberate policy not to discuss anything that was not seen as being fairly directly related to speech, and the nightmare episode was not considered as such. It was a research demand that this should be so, even though the ensuing dis-cussion might have been illuminating.

Session 27

Once again there is here an example of threat resulting in a relapse in speech the following week. The last comments of this session were:

L. To me it seems like this—if I was a fluent person, then it would be possible for me to do or say something which would mean somebody would certainly if not dislike me would wish to have nothing to do with me.
F. React unfavourably?
L. React unfavourably.

Session 28

The last session had ended with the discovery that one of the implications of being a fluent person is that one might do something that would make one disliked. But, of course, this idea has already met with considerable invalidation. When he has been fluent there has been no evidence that he has been disliked—he may even have thought people *liked* him! If he accepts that this superordinate construct has been invalidated, he would be faced with many other changes in his core role construing. If he is still not ready to do this he will return to stuttering. It is interesting that he himself links up his relapse with the idea of being disliked.

L. I think my speech has been getting worse ever since we started concentrating on 'being liked'. I have been thinking about ways in which one can get oneself disliked. I am becoming increasingly aware of just how mixed up I am, and what—or in fact, I want people to like me and in the past I've gone about getting them to like me in a certain way. Well, I am beginning to realize that the way I've gone about trying to get them to like me has had the exact opposite effect, and I'm left with absolutely nothing to cling onto to get people to like me except to stammer.
F. There is an alternative to your stammering, that is, people could actually like you *for yourself.*
L. [laughs] Yes—but of course—me—in people's eyes—up to this instance in time—me—is what I have been and if the me that was has tried to get people to like him using these means which I now realize have been having the opposite effect—then . . .
F. —there's a distinction between you *as a person* and you *in the way you behave?* You're describing behaviours that you adopt, aren't you?
L. Yes. But surely *'me' as a person* is seen by others as *'me' how I behave?*
F. That is true and I know what you mean. The minute you say you've been trying to get people to like you—this means you've been behaving in a way that is really not—that doesn't come naturally to you. In other words, it's being a 'not you'. Now I'm saying that still underneath that there's the person. And so, while you may not like the bit that makes you try to be liked—that's only one bit of you, and it's a false bit in your own eyes.
L. Yes . . .
F. We won't labour the point—we've been here before several times and surely all this is an indication of the direction in which you're moving.

L. Yes—I think it is—my wife said this last week—what she said was that my character is changing rapidly. She reckoned that in the past month or so it was beginning to change. She said in the past I used to be quite self-centred, and she said that I used to live in a little world of my own, but in the past month or so she has definitely noticed a change in this.

Quite clearly in this last excerpt there is an awareness of the change that is taking place within him. He is in a personal no man's land; he has had too much fluency to be a dedicated stutterer and not enough to be a really assured fluent speaker. So he clings, at the moment, to the idea that his stammer serves him as a protection. During the following three weeks interval he did some reconstruing that resulted in a further improvement in speech. This improvement continued, in fact, for the next fifteen weeks although with considerable fluctuation.

Session 29

L. I felt last week that I would have liked to have seen you because I was very conscious just what a bad inconvenient thing my stammer is and I felt that just a push in the right direction would have helped me along.

F. The fact that your speech improved suggests that you helped yourself a bit.

L. Yes. I certainly seem to have helped myself as far as my speech is concerned, but as far as my mental attitude is concerned I don't think I really have. What happened was—I began to realize that basically people do not like me when I stammer.

F. Was this based on observation?

L. Partly upon observation but mainly upon logical deduction. Because, after all, providing that all other things remain equal, it is far easier for a person to listen to and to understand someone who is fluent. And so I was very strongly aware of this feeling last week.

F. And this is a bit of a change for you?

L. Oh, yes, indeed, but this week I'm tending to slide back a bit and to think to myself 'well, perhaps people don't think I'm such a bad chap after all—and if I stammer a little they won't mind', and so I'm finding that this week my speech is pretty communicative, but it still has to have that hesitation and repetition which signifies a stammer.

He goes on to describe himself as a fluent person, and we then discuss this.

L. Last week I felt the need to give up stammering very strongly. This week I do not feel the need to give up quite so much.

F. Did this feeling of the need to give it up make you feel good, or depressed, or hopeful?

L. It made me feel good in a way, because I think that for the first time I could really imagine myself as a fluent person. I could not really imagine a situation in which I would stammer. But it also made me feel a little frustrated in that when anybody spoke I immediately started to think 'this—talking fluently —is so easy—why can't I?'

We then go on to discuss what this "fluent Luke" might be like.

L. I think that basically, whenever I'm a fluent person, I will still be as *kind*. I will still enjoy seeing other people happy as much as I do now—but I think I will have a far more *forceful* character.

F. Is that the same as strong?

L. Yes, I think it probably is. I think that probably at present my mind tends to link forcefulness of character with unpleasantness, or something like this.

F. Do you see yourself as joining these people who show their strength of character?

L. Yes I think I probably do. Things have happened during the last three or four months at work in which I've taken decisions or acted in ways which I thought were right and proper and which required considerable force and strength of character. I feel sure that in the past I would not have done these things.

Session 30

Once again we have the reiteration of the anxiety caused by the un-determined quality of the new "self", together with the unspoken thought that if he doesn't suffer fools gladly, maybe others will not suffer him gladly.

L. And so this chap was explaining it all again, and so I said 'it's all written down here, and I can read' or some acid like that which, looking back on it, probably was a little bit strong and was not really kind—but at the same time it was showing force, or strength of character.

F. Do you think such behaviour in such a situation is reasonable? That's the important thing, isn't it?

L. Well—yes—I . . .

F. Do you have to suffer fools gladly is the question, isn't it?

L Yes—well—I do not think one should have to, but I think that providing they do not get in one's way too much, one should put up with them, to a certain extent.

F. So, in fact, you're learning about being forceful.

L. Yes [laughs].

F. You're learning the limits of what is reasonable, and what's overdoing things and so on. If you've never acted in this way before, it's not surprising if you go too far from time to time. The thing is to modify your behaviour next time.

L. Yes.

F. What about being kind?

L. Well—I think that providing I do not go about biting other people's heads off all of the time, I think people will see me as a basically kind person. Because I think that I *am* a basically kind person.

F. It's taken us quite a time to get round to this, hasn't it? That the 'you' will shine through given half a chance.

L. Although I do not think that my character is probably a lot more forceful than I had at first thought. I think I will probably *have to be a little careful not to overdo things too much at first.*

These last two sessions are important because they indicate quite clearly the inherent dangers of being fluent and it was just such a condition that led to the relapse he experienced six months after the end of treatment. He discovered he *was* being too forceful—which meant being unpleasant—which meant not being liked—and so on. His reaction was to opt for the only other stance he knew, that of the stutterer.

Session 32

He returns now to the notion that "my stammer is disliked". Right at the end of this interview there is the remarkable statement that people will judge him by his fluency and not as a person.

L. The reason why my speech has been getting progressively worse during the past month is I think I realize that people are embarrassed when I stammer and so we've got this conflicting thing; the object of my stammer is to produce a favourable impression in people and, in fact, I'm realizing that's having the opposite effect.

F. You can't win . . .

L. I can't win [laughter].

F. That's a tough position to be in. What are you going to do about it?

L. Well—it would certainly seem that what has been happening is that my stammer has been getting worse and worse and worse. But, of course, this is a ridiculous thing. The other answer to this problem is a far more acceptable one—to talk fluently—but that seems at present to be just outside my grasp.

F. And yet you have these fantastic phases of fluency now.

L. Yes. I mean to say—this lunchtime I must have had a burst of fluency lasting maybe half an hour—of sensible conversation—talking about quite involved sorts of things.

F. Which I don't think you could have had in the past.

L. No.

*   *   *

L. You see, I am a different sort of person, but the thing is that the *majority of people will not measure my success in terms of this—they will measure my success in terms of fluency.*

During Session 15 Luke had discussed stuttering as being both a disguise *against* inadequacy and a sign *of* inadequacy. He is now opting for the latter. Stuttering gives an unfavourable impression which is probably of the general "weakness" type.

Session 33

In this interview Luke discovers another facet of fluent speech.

L. Today we were talking about something and we both said something at the same time. Well, up to now I would have stopped what I was saying in order to listen to what he was saying. But rather than doing that I continued to say what I wanted to say and my friend also said what he wanted to say and I found it was quite easy to say what I wanted to say but at the same time listen to what my friend said. And obviously my friend found exactly the same thing, because after he had finished saying what he wanted to say, he began to comment on what I'd just said!

F. What do you think about this?

L. I was quite surprised. I was not aware that one's attention could effectively be divided in two; some attention to speaking, some attention to listening. It was quite a new experience for me.

Right at the end he came back to the many imponderables of being fluent. He felt that a fluent person could say anything. For example, he could go up to anyone and say "what a big nose you have". Being fluent still is extremely threatening because it opens a new world of possible social interactions with which he feels he cannot deal. He was not convinced by the argument that social convention would make many of the decisions for him. His naïveté about fluency is still considerable. He is almost totally unaware of all the social rules of communication that operate to limit and guide speech. It is as if he sees fluency as a kind of essentially *uncontrolled* speech whereas he is aware of the *controlling* effects of stuttering.

The whole issue behind the present construct theory approach to stuttering is precisely this. A person sees meaning, control, predictive possibilities and organization as all implicitly bound up with stuttering (and perhaps other long-standing behavioural abnormalities), whereas, the alternative to stuttering (tics, asthma, hysterical reaction), which others would call "well", is essentially relatively a mysterious, uncontrolled, disorganized state of affairs.

Session 34

In this session he embarks on construing areas of communication such as problems of "openness", personal revelation and so forth, which are superordinate implications of *respect* and *liking*.

Session 38

He now construes communication at a subordinate level, concerning the rules of behaviour and elaborates at a superordinate level, formulated very vaguely right at the start, the idea of *pretending*; it now comes over in the form of *persuading* people:

L. I'm not necessarily asking you to give me a concise formula for persuading people, but just to give me some general ideas which I can develop myself to actually suit the situation—to suit my individual character . . .

F. One thing is to start observing how others do it.

L. Yes. I don't know. Whenever anybody does er persuading—either tries to persuade me or I hear somebody persuading somebody else, I immediately say to myself 'this person's trying to persuade me or is trying to persuade the other person'.

F. Is that bad?

L. Yes, I think it is.

F. Why?

L. I don't know really [laugh].
F. Surely it's all part of life and social interactions.
L. It does seem odd to me that somebody should effectively say to somebody 'all I'm saying now is just buttering you up so that you'll be persuaded'.

During this now very explicit elaboration of the idea of himself as a fluent speaker, he is implying that being persuasive would be out of character for him, it would be false flattery or *pretence* generally. In other words, for him stuttering is a kind of *honesty* and, if it were relinquished, it would have to be replaced by very simple direct speech which would have an equivalent "honesty". This superordinate construct of *honest* has hardly changed at all since he discussed it at the first session in spite of some fairly extensive elaborations in other parts of his system.

Session 39

Luke starts out by explaining a problem which relates exactly to what rather threatened him last time, namely, having to manipulate people by speech. He has advanced from his last position by arguing now that the end justifies the means—provided one's end is a "good" and "honest" one, it is permissible to use manipulation by speech to gain it.

F. Let us suppose there is a situation in which you want to get someone to do something for you. How would you go about it? What would you take into account?
L. I think the way I would go about this—the first question I'd ask would be 'is the end product a good and desirable thing?' If the answer is 'yes', then there would be reasons for it being a good and desirable thing and one should base one's persuasion or one's argument upon these reasons and provided the reasons are good, they cannot be broken. That is to say—one can logically say 'this is true—that is true—therefore the only obvious thing to do is to do this—and this is the end product'. OK. It also depends upon the person you're trying to persuade being a reasonable person and saying 'yes, I'll accept these as being reasonable reasons'. [laughter].

Session 40

This week's session followed a visit to his parents during which time his speech deteriorated. This is an example of the "movement interpretation of threat" described by Landfield (1954). A person will be seen as threatening if he expects the other "to be more like he used to be, or is now but no longer wants to be." In this case Luke's parents, unaware of any changes that have taken place in the ways he views life, expect him to be the same—a stutterer—as he has always been. Because of the expectancies of his parents and the resulting threat, he moves from uncertainty to certainty and again becomes the stutterer.

Session 41

Following this deterioration in speech as a result of the visit to the parents, there was a sudden improvement. It is possible that the threat-induced bad speech enabled him to perceive the degree to which he had changed. It offered him a chance of viewing the contrast and to realize that this was now no longer "him". He now moves on to make the most specific reference so far to construing of the other person's constructions.

F. The speaking situations you now find most difficult are the ones that are most difficult for the ordinary person.

L. I think this is so. Yes. I think that this is true. The sort of thing where one has to weigh up what the other person is thinking. If one's asking personal questions one has to decide whether or not they are offended, or likely to be offended. Or if you're explaining something you have to weigh up in your mind whether the person understands what you're talking about—this sort of thing . . .

The worst experience he reported as having had during the week was one in which he had to "sell" a job to someone who wasn't interested in it. He had to try and use his speech for manipulative purposes, directly and consciously. This indicates that *honesty* is still a construction to be reckoned with. The act of manipulating others has superordinate implications that eventually meet up and conflict with core role construing. He is, and wishes to be seen as, an honest man, but people who manipulate others are not behaving honestly. If he is fluent he may find he has to *persuade* and this makes fluency a threatening prospect.

This type of conflict may not be so uncommon among stutterers. Some forms of evaluative construction of the *honesty* type may be implicatively tangled up with the question of fluent speech, which would thereby make fluency a "bad thing" to achieve.

Through all the latest interviews he is continuing to construe the act of speaking fluently itself. On this occasion he is considering the use of silences. Previously, he has not been able to tolerate the idea that there will be any imperfections such as interjections or silences in his speech when he is trying to think up the words to use:

L. Certainly I don't like too long silences. There was a time when I wouldn't bring silences into my speech at all but I do now sort of stop in the midst of what I'm saying and am silent whilst I'm thinking—but I don't really know how long I can do this for—what is acceptable.

Session 42

The following speaks for itself:

L. The week before this was a *fantastically* good one . . . I think that the reason for my marked improvement was that I suddenly realized that I could not expect to be fluent in every situation—and—you know—at this present time—and from then on I was able to take confidence from the instances, from the times I was fluent in the easy situations. And also when I was not fluent in difficult situations, this did not upset me.

Session 43

We now come back to this problem of using speech to manipulate and persuade others. He starts off by telling of a shy young man who was unable to phone up the library and ask for some information even though he is fluent:

L. ... he is shy and, OK, he's fluent—but because he's shy or whatever it is he just cannot communicate and in this instance he probably suffers from more lack of communication than I do myself!

From the realization that people have difficulty in communicating with (manipulating) others, even though they are fluent, he goes on to tell of the mathematician he had to *persuade* to do a particular job and the difficulties he had in this *manipulation*. The whole superordinate construction of *honesty* is beginning to be elaborated, just as those to do with *respect* and status were.

Session 44

Luke has now advanced his construing of himself to the point where he admits, to some extent, that he is "living inside a shell or something". The truth of this is illustrated by the fact that when he thinks of having a conversation with his neighbour he can only think in terms of being interested in what the neighbour's job is. It is virtually only at this one fixed concrete level that he can think of interacting. Again, at the end of the session, there was concern about *persuasion*: this area of construing is still blocking progress, but at the moment he is unable to elaborate it more and work out its implications.

Session 45

In this interview Luke elaborates the notion of *pretence* by linking it with *conceit*. This, in turn, implies many of the aspects of *respect*. This linkage actually was stated as early as the first session.

L. I don't like to answer questions—I don't like to have to give a response I've never given before ... The problem is what is he going to think of me because of this reply I make? I think the problem here is lack of fluency in the past where one's—well—if one stammers then the fact that one stammers probably clouds everything else in the present—so my replies would have contained as few words as possible. Therefore they would be stinted of much content—other than necessities. And therefore it's been difficult for me to convey anything about my character in what I've said ... I'm very much afraid that people will think that I'm *conceited* or *big-headed*.

F. Do you think you are?

L. Um [silence]—no—I don't think so. I think that I am aware of my capabilities, and I don't believe in *pretending* to myself that I am not as good as I am, or something like that. But at the same time I don't pretend to myself that I'm better than I am . . .

Session 47

Constructs for the fourth NS-grid were elicited and laddered at this time.

In the previous interview Luke asked his first real favour and found, to his intense surprise, that he was not only able to do it, but to do it fluently. Instead of thinking to himself that it was a favour, he thought he was simply asking for something to be done and that was quite justifiable. It seems more likely that this experience and the consequent elaboration of his system that must have accompanied it, led to the following reply when asked to state the opposite of someone who stutters.

L. The opposite of stuttering. [prolonged silence] I can see what could happen here though. In the past I've been looking at it from a purely physical point of view —a stutterer is someone who hesitates in his speech. I feel that I'd like to bring in something new which also includes the mental outlook as well. Can I put down a physically *and mentally* fluent person?

He has thus put himself right up against the implications of the fluency pole of stuttering/fluency construct, by placing a considerable extension of its range of convenience and its type of implications into the "psychological" sphere.

Sessions 48, 49, 50

Constructs for the fourth S-grid were elicited and laddered and the grids administered during this time.

The next three interviews are rather impoverished. They concentrate on rather factual aspects of communication such as details of holding conversations rather than on the people holding them. In the 50th interview, there seems to be an awareness of this on Luke's part.

L. . . . Because, presumably, if I did happen to level off, you/we could have some quite deep and serious conversations to sort out the cause.

'Deep and serious conversations' presumably refer to some more elaborate and superordinate construing that we had been doing previously.

Session 51

Things are on the move again. Luke initiates a discussion of relationship between fluency and his job ambitions. Particularly the fact that fluency would involve him in putting other constructions to the test, such as his abilities to rise in his career, and that these might prove invalid.

Session 52

In this interview he goes on to explore the interpersonal implications of stuttering and fluency in relation to his job ambitions. At the end he again comes round to *pretence*, this time in the guise of 'talking down' to people. It is almost as if, were he modest and introverted on the one hand or extraverted and aggressive on the other, he would subsume them both under the "pretence" end of a *pretence–genuine* construct.

> L. One friend is a fantastic extravert—he's so proud and conceited and he's good fun—and he is extremely successful. And when he comes round and visits us, we always have a laugh when he goes, because he's so—so extravert and conceited. And I feel that probably if I was being my true self I'd be something like that as well—and I also feel that when I get marked bouts of fluency—I don't just mean ordinary sorts of fluency, but *marked* bouts of fluency—I am becoming very much like this . . .
>
> You know—I sort of get—I haven't really come to terms with this yet—this feeling of—if I became more extravert and a little more conceited and a little more of a show-off, or something—sort of get the feeling people are going to say 'who does he think he is?' . . . How can I just be a little extraverted and guard against going to this extreme.
>
> F. Surely all this is relative? You are experiencing the freedom of fluency and are taking a pleasure in talking.
>
> L. Yes, I think that is probably correct because when I had that spell of good fluency recently I thought that I was probably being quite extraverted but my wife said how much more confident I seemed—and everybody thought that I was more confident. So whereas I thought I was doing a bad thing I was in fact doing a good thing.

Session 54

In the previous session, Luke had given a fairly faithful reiteration of the Johnson's aetiological theory of stuttering which had, in turn, been discussed with him at various stages in his treatment. By doing this he shows how he now accepts a truly explanatory theory of his stuttering as opposed to the early days when he either offered no theory or a simple tautology like 'it's caused by anxiety'. He now provides an elaboration of his own. He argues that because the child cannot eliminate his stutter, he exaggerates it in order to obtain sympathy instead of parental criticism. He argues further, that this process may operate in some similar, although presumably more elaborate, way in adult life. However, Luke seems to have difficulty in carrying this on further to the whole question of the implications of "getting sympathy" and how this may be the background meaning of his desire for liking, for status, for respect, and so forth; and how this, in turn, may lead to an emphasis on honesty, pretence and genuineness.

L. I have been thinking about this sort of thing in general terms and I'm sort of slowly devising a theory. It isn't put together particularly well yet and I've not really collected and analysed my ideas to form a whole. But if you would care to just hear what—basically it sort of works like this: that a child is told to talk properly or something like this and this concentrates the child's attention on his speech and also gives the child the feeling that it is wrong to talk incorrectly. And probably the child doesn't really know what's meant by talking properly because he probably thinks he's talking all right anyway. And so you get built up 'it is nasty and wrong to stammer, people will not like you if you stammer'—sort of thing—in child language. Now the child doesn't know what to do about this, but because of the parents' attention to hesitations in speech, which I think it is at that stage, and probably the attention of the friends of the parents to this as well—because the parents have discussed it—and because of the reaction of the friends—a sort of sympathetic reaction almost—the child is doing something he can't help. It's like a lame or blind child. They give him sympathy. The child soon realizes, and probably the parents as well are—tend to vacillate between trying to punish the child for disfluencies and also trying to—rather than punishment—reward him for fluency perhaps or then again perhaps try sympathy—just a general 'not knowing what to do' on behalf of the parents. The child soon catches on that if, in fact, he makes his disfluency severe—and this is the important thing—he will gain overall sympathy. And I think that this is the sort of basis of it—a little disfluency—the parents sort of say 'this is wrong—don't talk like this because it sounds silly'—a severe disfluency sounds absolutely horrible and they don't think it's silly but it's really pitiful.

F. 'Poor child.'

L. The child is told, or is told to get rid of imperfections in its speech—it doesn't know how to get rid of the imperfections but it does know how to get rid of being told to stop these imperfections—and I think it probably goes something like that.

F. So why does the child go on doing it?

L. It goes on doing it because it cannot get rid of this imperfection because it has opted to sort of effectively get rid of punishment by making the imperfection worse. But all the child has done is remove the punishment shall we say. But there is still this imperfection there and the child must surely realize that even though the parents don't say it in so many words 'stop this now'—it realizes that this imperfection is an undesirable thing. But it is less undesirable than the punishment for it—the minor imperfections—and the thing is—I think that this also builds up in the child this feeling of a need to be perfect in his speech.

*   *   *

L. The child's way out is not for his stammer to be improved but for it to be worse. And I think the same thing happens to me. The only way I know of getting out of an uncomfortable situation, as far as my stammer's concerned, is to make it worse.

Session 56

In the early part of this interview Luke makes a general plea for simplicity in his construing of relationships with other people. This indicates his present awareness of the complexities that are continually arising as the stuttering ceases to dominate. In the past, the stutter, in itself, has simplified the interpersonal speaking situation for him. In further discussing personal interactions we are inevitably drawn into discussions of *status*. But now there is continued evidence of the extension of previous construing in that his reactions are related to the *relative* status of the person to whom he is talking.

L. In one situation I put myself below the person in order to appease him, or something like this. It does sound a bit odd but I think this is something of the sort of thing that does happen—the criticism situation—I'm in a position in which I'm happily below the other person in status.

F. Do you *mean* happily below?

L. Um. I don't think I do. Acceptably—no—um—no—such as our relationship then—I don't feel that I want to assert myself in any way.

F. Yes, but should you wish to put over a point . . .

L. Yes, exactly. Then I come up against this problem.

F. And is it then that you push yourself happily below in status? This enables you to say 'I have no right to criticize'. If you are an equal you have a right.

L. Yes, indeed. When I said happily having lower status, I don't mean consciously happy—you know . . .

F. It sounds rather like "resignedly"—or . . .

L. No. It's just something which has been sorted out by the subconscious and it's not—I've not really thought about it myself—I think that actually this problem happens a lot to my relationships with people. That I—without thinking—put myself in an inferior position to them.

F. Which would mean that this limits your social interaction with them.

L. Yes. Certainly I don't put myself in a position where I could assert myself so far as they're concerned [said dreamily and almost doubtfully].

Perhaps if he felt he could assert himself he would overdo it and they would say 'who does he think he is'.

L. I think there is something in my mind which I'd like to try to say. I can't quite put my finger on it [long silence]—I think it is—if one adopts an inferior role would one sort of assume less responsibility . . .

F. For what?

L. For things. [laughs]—I'm talking rather abstractly—vaguely—no—I think my concepts about all this are so vague that I would like to take time to think about them.

He is becoming increasingly adept at thinking loosely, but imposes limits on how much will be said aloud. However, a little later on he continues, asserting oneself changes to a discussion of *showing-off* by using unusual words.

L. Yes, of course—I think that actually this is—I think that we're back to this status thing again. Yes. So then, if, say, I use these rather fine words to somebody, I've put myself on equal position, then that person is, basically, if I put myself on equal position with somebody then in fact that person is probably inferior to me—and so . . .

F. Sorry—I haven't quite followed that.

L. Because I set my position as, say, one step down from where it should be—if I set my position as being equal with somebody—in fact—I'm one step up . . . I am trying to formulate two different situations in which I would feel uncomfortable about saying the same thing. The first situation I am inferior to the person I am talking to and I am trying to bring myself up level and in the other position I would be level or superior in which case by saying it I would be showing-off.

F. Not if you were level—why are you . . .

L. Because if I considered myself to be level I would probably realize that in fact I am superior [laughter]

F. You're going to make sure you win, aren't you? [laughter]

L. No. OK then. Let us formulate three situations—the one where I am inferior and I would be trying to bring myself up; the second situation where I am exactly equal and it has no effect at all and would be said fluently; and the other situation where I would be showing-off.

Session 57

The whole of this session is taken up with Luke's continued efforts to elaborate his construing of status. In spite of considerable elaboration having already taken place, the concept is still very undeveloped and it is not surprising that it still gives him so much trouble. Whereas it seems likely that most people have at least three constructs of status *superior–inferior, superior–equal, inferior–equal,* Luke seems only to have *superior–inferior.* Though he uses the word 'equal', it does not really seem to be an actual operating distinction. He can only use *status* in some superordinate global sense and does not see it as situational, related to areas of construing, related to moral qualities and so forth.

Session 59

With the status dilemma still unresolved, Luke comes back to the question of rules for fluency—what should he do in particular situations. When it is pointed out that this has nothing to do with stuttering, he agrees, but says that the only way he could give up stammering permanently would be by knowing all the rules of fluency. He then carries out an experiment with emphasizing words.

L. Now, I am deliberately experimenting with emphasizing what I am saying—and it seems to be working alright. I seem to be talking fluently now. This is something else I have been bothered about. I feel I have a very monotonous sounding voice.

By replaying the recording of his use of emphasis he agrees that it sounded perfectly all right. We go on.

L. One interesting thing you mentioned just now, when I was emphasizing my words, you said that my voice sounded much more assertive.
F. Yes. I'm not too sure that is the right word.
L. I think it is. I *felt* a lot more assertive as well. I don't know which comes first because when I was emphasizing my words I was talking fluently and I wonder if it was in fact the emphasis that I was putting on my words that was causing fluent speech or whether it was the fact that I was feeling assertive what I am trying to say which gave me confidence.

The discussion shows that he is beginning to *use* constructs which have a range of convenience covering both voice tone and manner as well as psychological implications and relationships with other people.

Session 60

In many of the interviews, Luke seems to be saying the same thing over and over again, and, for practical purposes, in many cases he is. However, it is very easy to mistake the construct for its verbal label. In some cases it is obvious from the context and the way he is working things out, that he is really seeing a new aspect to the elements about which he is talking. For example, looked at superficially, the notion of being *relaxed* in the following passage seems to be exactly the same point he has already made many times before in relation to notions like confidence. But it seems clear from the context that he is, from his own point of view, elaborating his interpretation of what goes on inside the speaker in relation to how he speaks and other aspects of communication. It is very easy to under-rate the degree of elaboration which a person is achieving when he doesn't signal it clearly by using very new and striking verbal labels. It may sound very circular and repetitive from the listener's point of view.

L. I feel that this property of being relaxed in situations is terrifically important, isn't it? I suppose the thing is that stammerers are always conscious of themselves, aren't they? And conscious of not only everything that they say, but everything that they do, the general effect that they are having on other people and the influence they are having on others. I think that for a long time I have been conscious of what people do and what people say, but I don't think that I have really had anything to apply it to. I've been studying, for example, the way in which one person communicates with another. But because I don't communicate with anybody, I've not had the occasion to apply it. And things that are not applied are soon forgotten.

Session 61

For more than ten days he has been experiencing his best speech so far, but says that 'it is definitely a very nice situation to be in, but also a rather frightening sort of situation, certainly a situation that provokes some excitement. I don't mean happy excitement'. I ask if he is aware of a fundamental change.

L. I think I would go as far as saying a fundamental change. I felt previously when I stammered, when I did something or thought something and people didn't agree, I had to find an excuse for holding this point of view. Now the thing that has taken the time to realize, and it may sound silly, but it is that I must hold these views for good reasons and all I have to do is find these reasons for holding these views and defend them. I was a little on the timid side and ready to accept other people's views but I am defending my own views now and this is something I never did before and I think it is a fundamental change.

F. In a way you are being more 'you'.

L. Yes, yes. I don't know why I should have been like that. I suppose it must hinge on wanting to say as little as possible. It's far easier to back down and say I was probably wrong. I rather wonder how long this fluency is going to last. I have a sort of fear about it.

F. Remember, you have never had this sort of experience in your life before.

L. Yes, it's quite a thing really isn't it. Quite exciting really.

F. So it is no good asking how long it is going to last. For having experienced it you can never go right back.

L. I've suddenly thought of an argument which is better, which makes me quite happy again. The argument is that it is a good thing to have bad spells, because at least these bad spells do stand out and you can look at them and find out the cause of them, so if I relapse it will be a good thing. It will mean that there is still something else to be talked about and it should be easy to discover what it is. Whereas if I continue to have the sort of fluency I have now there is still something left to discover, but my speech is so uniformly good it would be difficult to find it. Looking at it from that point of view, I think that it will make one tend to look forward to one's relapses.

During the next week he continued to improve and starts off in the next session by voicing some doubts.

Session 62

F. So, what is life like now?

L. Well it is very interesting. What I wanted to talk to you about was—I suppose now I am starting to find my true character and I think I am finding I have a very forceful character. What I am wondering about is how does forcefulness— no is it possible for people to have a forceful character and still be nice people? Liked by people?

F. What makes you think they can't be?

L. I don't know. I just think that I am going to be the type of person who wants his own way you see. Now I had assumed that people don't or at least didn't exceptionally like people who want their own way.

* * *

F. Has this been a fear at the back of your mind for some time, how people would react?

L. I don't think so. I think it is purely the sort of thing of not how people would react to me as a forceful person, but just how people would react to me as a fluent person. What do I sound like when I am fluent? Do I say the right things?

F. And you find . . . ?

L. Yes. Perfectly all right. I've also been a little apprehensive in the change in myself. This is the first time I'm going to be fluent and so it is something new. I rather like being a forceful type of person and I think even when I stammered I used to try to be forceful or at least as forceful as I could, it was part of me even then.

In the doubts that Luke expressed about himself *vis-à-vis* fluency, he demonstrates the three quite different levels of construing around which he circles. At the most subordinate level he is concerned with the implications of fluency for the actual mechanisms of speech, questions of tone, emphasis and so forth. At another level of abstraction, he is concerned with the implications of fluency, for the whole business of conversation and subjects and acceptability of different topics and how to keep the conversation going and so forth. At the highest level of abstraction he is concerned with the implications of fluency for his whole character, his whole relationship to other people in his life, his core role constructs.

The next five sessions are concerned with discussions of personal relationships at work. With his new-found fluency, he talks openly of 'manipulating' people and at no time does he manifest any difficulty with the whole idea of persuasion and its "bad" moral implications that so bothered him in earlier interviews. There is a general picture of a man pushing forward to be an individual, developing his own life along the path he himself dictates. He can be clearly seen groping outwards in an attempt to relate his major area of construing, which is centred on his job, to other aspects such as interpersonal relationships, and to develop constructs such as *articulate* and *authoritative*, which might have a range of convenience covering both areas. In Session 67, there seemed to be very little for either participant to say. As Luke "runs out" of stuttering, the interviews become more and more impoverished as personal problems unrelated to speech are not considered valid topics of discussion in a research context.

During this period of time the fifth NS- and S-grids were completed. In the NS-grid the self construct was related in a massive way with many constructs particularly those concerned with interpersonal relationships. The S-grid was grossly impoverished by comparison. It can be argued that such a tightly-knit, monolithic structure as that of the NS-grid is fragile—it can brook no modification, it has no flexibility.

Session 68

In this he gives an example of feedback about his fluency which was clearly very helpful to him.

L. I don't know if you remember when I was very worried about assembling my thoughts, arguing and bringing pertinent points to bear, I mentioned a person who I thought was fairly good at this. The interesting situation was that we were trying to do some work and went across to visit some accountants. I took this man with me because he would do this work. The next day he said what a difficult sort of conversation that was. He said 'I wonder what they could have thought of me yesterday afternoon, I just sat and said nothing at all. It's a very vague sort of conversation the type of thing when one is turning over thoughts and really I think it must be very difficult to conduct the conversation so that you are continually bringing the other people out, keeping them talking, directing them in this way'. I said 'yes, I think it must be very difficult' and he sort of looked a bit funny, and I thought and I said to him, 'just a minute, do you mean that you thought I had conducted the conversation like that' and he said 'yes'. I was so amazed and said 'that's interesting', because he said 'it must take a lot of practice to be able to do this'. I was completely unaware of this, unaware of the difficulty of the situation.

Session 69

This, and the following three sessions were conducted at the "technical" level of abstraction. This continual search for rules is very reminiscent of the way a young adolescent feels about the whole business as he starts to move on towards sociality. The young adolescent often feels that there must be some set rules, some known principles, some relatively simple and sure-fire techniques for doing these things (how to win friends and influence people). It is as if the stutter had prevented Luke from maturing conversationally at all, so that as his stutter begins to fade, he finds himself in the position of, say, a fifteen year old who is trying to spread his conversational wings.

General discussion next focused on the actual words on which he now stutters. The common denominator is agreed to be "emotionally-loaded" words and "status-loaded" words. It is almost as if the sessions had come round a full circle, only now these are the only words giving trouble, whereas before the presence of these words triggered off stuttering on most of the other words. Reminiscent of earlier times also is this statement:

L. I think there are two situations—there is a situation where I genuinely want to get on well with people—then there is the other situation where I really am being insincere because all that I'm after is to either butter them up or to establish a good relationship—whether that—you know what I mean—or to get my way or something like that.

He goes on to experiment with verbal skills which go beyond the ability simply to use speech generally, to the level at which he can play around with the very conventions of speech themselves.

L. There is a chap who is quite prepared to pull people's legs and sort of jokingly say things against a person. And I find that I can use these status-loaded words against him far better than anybody else. I feel that he is more happy about the status situation—and I can use very erudite words against him and I let them roll off my tongue with real pleasure and satisfaction. And I know he realizes in this case I'm using them purely as a battering ram against him really and it's the sort of thing which he quite enjoys. So it seems to me that the problem that I have is being able to use these words in an enjoyable way to people who might take offence—or at least whom I feel might be offended.

F. I think that's fair enough—although I don't see why it should make you stammer. One doesn't want to try to use these words with everybody does one?

L. That's fair enough. I suppose that perhaps what I may have been getting at but didn't realize was that with this person, one used them specifically as a status symbol—as a battering ram—as a verbal weapon to reply to his verbal barrage. It wouldn't exactly be an onslaught, but the thing is that in other situations where one uses these status-loaded words in the specific context because one really wants to use them in all their meaning and not for their status-loaded implication. There's the fear that people will think that you're not using them for their meaning but for their status-loaded implications—an attempt to sort of 'batter' them.

Session 73

At the beginning of this session he goes straight on talking about emotionally and status-loaded words. This leads him into a long speech in which he makes a real attempt to review and overview his present situation. He has got it centred down to core role construing in the question of *me–not me*. The difficulty seems to be that, just as he had at one time an oversimplified construction of *stuttering–fluency* so that fluency was a kind of simple perfect speech, so now, in a sense, he has an oversimplified construct *me–not me*. Being *me* is an exact and simple expression of his feeling at the time. He has no more elaborate constructions that can take care of long term as opposed to short term events or *me* in relation to this person as opposed to that person and so forth. In attempting to overview, he specifically makes a comparison with *me* six or seven years ago, which is a kind of superordinate construction that he has not previously used very much.

L. Let's try and analyse it [the remaining stutter]. It's definitely caused by the relationship between myself and somebody else. This is very general, and the fact that I want to maintain a good relationship with this person. In other words, this person is sufficiently important, this person is somebody who I *want* to maintain a good relationship with. This doesn't apply to everybody. And in how I say a thing I am afraid that will affect this good relationship, probably because I don't know what reaction the other person will have toward what I say or . . .

F. What do you guess?

L. I usually guess that they are going to react unfavourably, because if I guess they will be favourable the situation does not bother me. So obviously my past experience is that people react to certain things that I have said in a way that I would not expect them to, and if at times people have reacted unfavourably to things I have said—which I could see no reason why they should—yes, probably I think that really one of the troubles I had a few years ago, quite a long time ago five or six years, I tried, I used to say—I used to say what a clever sort of person I thought I was. I thought people would realize that I was trying to make a joke, but they didn't and they thought I was conceited or something else. You see it took a very long time for me to realize this, because in the days when I stammered quite a lot I was completely, you know, as we discussed some time ago—I was not aware of people's cues. And so I would say a thing and their reaction to it would not really get through. They would be silent or something, but silence did not really mean anything and really when I realized that people took me at my word that rather shocked me. Probably this is something I have not quite got over, that if you are not careful people you know will take one—will in fact read into things meanings that have not been meant. Indeed, this I think was a very disturbing thing especially when I started very badly and I more or less forced myself to say it so that there was no possibility of deviation and if people read a meaning into my sentence which probably was constructed to contain words that I knew I could say easily and therefore was probably a strangely constructed sentence, and was wide open to having different meanings read into it. I think that this disturbed me quite a bit really. And I am still not happy about saying things to people and being afraid they are going to read some other meaning into it. Now I don't think this is really all the problem. Here we have the relationship between myself and somebody else and I am saying something and on the basis of what I am going to say they are going to have an unfavourable reaction. This unfavourable reaction is what they read into what I say. The other situation about this time I was talking about five or six years ago, there were people I had to ask to do things and that and I remember once someone got really angry with me when I asked them to do things. They sort of said that one should ask people to do things and not *order* them to do things—you see I did not understand this. Certainly here again was a situation when I was asking someone to do something in a reasonable way. It was not my intention to order them, but they took this attitude about it, and I think it is this that I have got left over. I don't want to order people around. I don't want people to think that I am conceited. I don't want people to have unfavourable reactions to me and I am not happy that what I am saying satisfies these criteria. I think that this is probably now getting fairly close to the root of this thing which is producing the difficulties that I am having.

To help him continue this extensive verbalization of these varied constructions, I asked him to tell me what the differences are between the "him" six years ago and the "him" now.

L. I suppose that the major difference is that I would hope to be able to say the things that I want to say, rather than commit myself to a sentence. Now again, another disadvantage of six years ago was that having said something and really felt it was wrong, it was a terrible strain to say something else to try to get out of the situation. I would hope that I would be better at doing that now.

But I feel that the influence of my past is still with me, in that it does not come to my mind to try and get myself out of a situation that I have made a mess of. It does not come to mind. My immediate reaction is to stay quiet and say nothing more in case I get in deeper. In the same way my reaction is to stutter. I haven't got this switch. So the differences between me now and six years ago is that now I would hope to be in a better position to be more flexible about what I say and to be more able to get myself out of a situation by use of speech. I should be more fluent and proficient in my use of speech, which, indeed I really am. But I don't feel that the instinct is there. I suppose if the instinct was there I would be a fluent person.

F. Yes. And you are asking a bit much in hoping it comes overnight.

L. I do find that when these things come they come very quickly. Indeed, when they come I think they have been there all the time.

F. Isn't another big difference that speaking now gives an indication of 'you', whereas six years ago speaking gave no indication of you.

L. Yes. Yes. You see as soon as you say that, what comes into my mind is a feeling of the situation in which I am not showing 'me'. I'm trying to keep this good relationship—it's rather a bad way of putting it, but I feel that I am not really being 'me'. I say 'if you're not too busy would you mind doing this'. It's not really me. It's me trying to be nice; me trying to keep up this good relationship; me trying not to order someone about. I think the crux of the matter was that although I was, say, accused of ordering people about, I have never really understood it. I have never really understood why. I don't know what constitutes ordering people about. I am trying to avoid doing something I don't really understand.

This view, that we should only do or say things we really feel, is a restatement of the *genuine–honesty* idea and indicates a still unelaborated system for construing interpersonal relationships. During the course of this session an idea was discussed about "letting the subconscious do the talking for you".

The discussion was aimed at using this *genuine* construct to invalidate the restricting notion that there are specific rules governing speech in particular and communication in general.

In this following session, he sees the discussion on the subconscious as the most significant aspect of the entire session. He sees the significance of the idea of naturalness or spontaneity in speech and how it, in turn, is a rejection of his previous notion of there being rules for conversation which he ought to learn. At a deeper level the acceptance of this is almost a reversal of his life's style, which seems to be generally very restricted and unflowing.

Session 74

L. I think I may really be on the improvement again. When I plotted my past week's results and I saw this improvement again—for the very first time since I have done it—I thought, 'thank goodness, I'm improving again'. Previous times I looked at it and I had rather a start to notice that I was suddenly going to get better or rather than they were taking downward trends. And this was the first time I did not have a little start of fright.

F. When did it happen, this drop?

L. It seemed to date from the last time I saw you. We had quite a deep discussion and I went away feeling quite a bit happier.

F. Can you think of something specific we discussed.

L. I think it was this thing I mentioned about letting the subconscious do the talking for you. I remember I felt a certain easing of this problem I had had of being *artificial*, or at least saying things I thought I should say rather than things I really felt I should say.

The extent to which he now construes himself as a stutterer is revealed in the next excerpt. He is not quite ready to relinquish the idea.

F. You still stammer?

L. Um [long pause] I suppose I don't really—I suppose I just hesitate.

F. Are you still a stammerer?

L. Um I am still disfluent because it depends how you define the word stammerer. If you define a stammerer as a person who has disfluencies in his speech because of some quite major psychological disturbance, then I don't think I am a stammerer, but if you define a stammerer purely as someone who has disfluencies in his speech, then I am one.

F. You have never found it necessary to make this distinction before.

L. Haven't I? No. [laugh]

F. If I had asked you six months ago you wouldn't have hesitated in your answer I think.

L. No. I think I was trying to make it in the last couple of tests we have done, the Impgrids, but the—but I don't think I got as far as mentioning psychological disturbance.

F. If someone came to you and said 'you are a stammerer, aren't you', would you have to hesitate before giving an answer?

L. I um I don't really know. If someone said 'I know you are a stammerer' I wouldn't contradict them, but if they said 'are you a stammerer?'—yes, that's it—I would probably say 'I used to be but I am just in the process of overcoming it' or something like that.

F. You still feel it necessary to qualify your answer.

L. Yes, I think that there are times when I think I do more than hesitate on a word, when there is a blockage or repetition on a word that is more than a hesitation, and these words crop up unexpectedly, or unexpectedly for me.

Session 75

Many months before, Luke was confused about his role in society as a scientist, how he was in doubt about his role as a fluent speaker who will be *seen to be* a 'superior educated person'—how he was not the sort of person who *should* be fluent. His concern with status is now very much in relation to himself as a fluent person. The solution of his stuttering problem has raised for him all kinds of new problems in the sense that people's range of action in relation to himself has vastly increased.

L. Yes—I have a feeling you know that this little bit of trouble I've got left is still a status-loaded thing. As I become fluent—as I become more and more fluent, more and more proficient with my speech, I'm going to become more and more clever—can you see what I'm trying to get at?

F. Yes.

L. And I wonder whether I'm going to be happy about people's reaction to me being so clever and so articulate . . .

F. Well—what sort of reactions are you expecting—or fearful of?

L. I think we might well be going back to this 'big-headed' thing again—or a status-loaded thing. I'm going to become more and more articulate and therefore more and more respected because of my true intelligence. My true ability is going to become more and more apparent. Well now, I think—that's interesting —I think that perhaps what's happening is this then: supposing that originally I was at this place on the social scale, or respect scale or whatever have you, high social value, respected, very clever—this sort of thing—I was a stammerer and I was there perhaps [pointing to a chart]. I knew where I fitted. I have now become more fluent and I'm moving up to there. But I'm but the process of moving along there meant a continual—has meant me continually accepting my new position—accepting that the people—or at least being happy that people accept me in that position. So I wonder if what has happened is not a complete removal of this respect thing—a complete cure of this respect thing— but just that I have accepted my new position in life. And I wonder if now, with absolute fluency and being able to become quite—to be able to be quite articulate, my position's going to rise even more. Now what's happened is that I'm not sure about people's reactions to me in this position—new position. So I wonder if perhaps there is still something in this respect line that has not been cured but has been side-stepped because, rather than digging it out by its roots and chopping all the roots and throwing it away, we put weed-killer on it and it's shrivelled away or it's been accepted but the roots are still there . . . Yes—Perhaps the big-head thing isn't a very good way of describing it although what I'm worried about is people—silly isn't it? People seeing me as a superbly articulate person and thinking—'ah, but the upper-classes are usually the most articulate'—as I'm saying this I realize what absolute nonsense I'm talking!

F. Fair enough. I can't see . . .

L. This is the type of thing I feel that is in my mind. The fact that I still cannot see it—or at least I can see it with my mind but I can't feel it, something like that— I cannot feel that I am anything but—I cannot feel myself as being a superior, educated person . . .

F. No, because you'd call that inferiority—equality—or something.

L . Yes, perhaps so—I can't see myself—I can't *feel* myself the type of person who should be articulate . . .

F. Well, that's not surprising as you haven't been articulate for the whole of your life. I really must argue with you surely about the upper-classes being articulate, because they are among the most inarticulate [laughter] imaginable. The other thing I wanted to say was about 'respect' and being possibly disrespected for being articulate. Surely it depends—if one is able to express oneself well—surely respect depends on how much you respect the other person. Now if you respect the listener, or the people you're talking to you will treat them accordingly. You won't talk down to them or you won't do any of the things that you *could* do as an articulate person.

L. Yes [grudgingly] OK—I think that probably I mean something slightly different to this. It's not—or at least what I'm worried about is not what I'm going to say to the other person—and talking down to them or anything like this—what I'm worried about is that just in talking naturally but articulately—even to other people—supposing I'm talking to A, talking away and B happens to be listening, the thing which worries me—I think I'll exaggerate it a bit to make it very non-sensical and very obvious—that I suppose—yes—that B is going to be jealous or in fact envious, or at least B is going to be—or say to himself 'oh, that chap talks very well, he's using jolly good words—the correct words in the correct context—yes—he talks jolly well—what right has he got to be talking so well—he's only a so-and-so'.

F. [laughter] No, you don't really—I don't really believe you think that. OK, there may be envy but there's nothing wrong about envy in most people. I'm envious of all sorts of people. But in a way you respect people more if you envy them.

L. Oh yes, I don't mind people envying me because, as you say, this is something which is a compliment to oneself.

F. If you're really going to worry about the twisted person who turns round and says 'what right has he got to be born like this?'—which is fundamentally what you're saying . . .

L. Ah—but—*I* am the twisted person who is thinking that that person is saying that.

F. OK. But you are thinking about a twisted person—so if you two twisted people want to get together—OK [laughter]—there's nothing you can do if a person does think that—because it's a totally unusual and abnormal thing to think.

Session 82

This was the last interview to be taped, and occurred eight months after Session 75. The intervening monthly sessions became more and more impoverished with regard to content, more and more concerned with general events. This was because Luke was becoming increasingly confident about himself as a fluent, articulate person and it was thought desirable to allow him to consolidate this view of himself at his own speed.

At this session he reports a conversation he had with someone who had given a paper at a conference:

L. A paper was presented by somebody else which I was very interested in—and I buttonholed him afterwards—and asked a few points and I did it really without thinking. And I afterwards realized that I just hadn't stammered at all. It had come so naturally to go up to a stranger and sort of catch hold of his arm so that he would turn round and say 'I enjoyed your paper, there are one or two things I wanted . . .' you know.

F. This must have seemed very important to you.

L. I think it definitely was. I definitely didn't realize I was doing it. I didn't realize the *enormity* of what I was doing—when I did it. But I realized it afterwards. And it's interesting really, because there I was talking away fluently—and after being there a couple of days the enormity of it was just too much for me and I went into a restaurant and asked for a cup of coffee—I just had to stammer a little!

Six Months Later

Tightly-knit, unidimensional construct systems as that shown on the fifth NS-grid are vulnerable if one of the superordinate constructs receives invalidation. Such systems have little flexibility. Every invalidating breeze rustles the implications throughout.

Invalidation on a massive scale is what Luke experienced and it not surprisingly produced conceptual chaos to do with "being a fluent person". This, in turn, made him seek for a meaningful way of relating to people. He returned to stuttering.

The massive invalidation was a sudden realization that his newly adopted life-style was unacceptable to him. He did not like the *aggressive, forceful* person he perceived himself to be. That there had been considerable change in his construing can be seen from the fact that he did not report that *others* did not seem to like him, but just that he did not like *himself*.

The superordinate lines of implication of the construct *aggression* had never been properly sorted out. He had not been able to disentangle the question that fluency might mean aggressiveness, which might mean being a "bad" person. So, when he moved into fluency, he was suddenly brought up against a picture of himself which was not a workable, acceptable one from his point of view. By contrast, in the case of the construct *honest*, he had been able to see that fluency did not necessarily mean dishonesty. He was able to go ahead and be fluent without colliding with that aspect of his evaluative core role constructions.

Gradually, over many months (during which time he attended at three or four weekly intervals) he returned to his former level of fluency.* This was achieved by discussing the central idea that our personality characteristics are not construed on an all-or-none basis. It is all right to be *forceful* in certain situations, downright *aggressive* in others and submissive or gentle in others. The roles we adopt towards people are dependent upon the ways in which we construe the construction processes of the other. From putting our case over forcibly in the first instance, we may change to being sympathetic to the other's problems as we see him wavering towards accepting our point of view.

B. GENERAL COMMENTS

The treatment of Luke's stutter, his subsequent relapse and the reinstatement of his fluency, covered more than four years. A long time by most standards. That this is not solely a function of the treatment procedure is shown by the fact that many of the group improved markedly in months rather than years.

* Since the completion of the analysis of disfluencies ,Luke has continued to increase his level of fluency; there now being less than one disfluency per 100 words.

To a large extent the period of time needed to bring about any change in Luke's construing system was the result of the extreme impoverishment of his interpersonal constructions. It is more than possible that any one, stutterer or not, who was so at sea in the world of other humans would have needed, or at least benefited from, some form of help. Looking back on his former self, he agrees that he was very "mixed up" and that this is now not the case. He feels much more certain of himself, and that most of his interpersonal problems have been ironed out. One only remains—he is not yet confident of his ability to "make a good job" of relating to people. He is not absolutely convinced that they will not misunderstand him and his motives. A period of sixteen weeks between improvements to new levels of fluency is considerable. Whether this speed was determined by the resistance of his system to change or to my taking him at too slow a rate there is no way of knowing (see Figs. 19 and 20).

The improvement in his social competence was brought about by concentrating on the implicative networks surrounding certain superordinate constructs and attempting to look at the evidence he used to validate his predictions. It was often the case that he "extorted validational evidence" (showed hostility in the Kellian sense) since validating evidence was clearly not there. By working away at the subordinate implications of these superordinate constructs, such as those to do with status, respect, and honesty, it was hoped to show him enough invalidation to persuade him to modify the system, eventually up to and including the superordinate level.

One point raised by this therapeutic approach concerns the time at which treatment should be terminated. Because of the form of the research, topics outside those connected with speech itself, taken in its widest meaning, were not considered valid areas for discussion. For this reason, as fluency increased, so topics to discuss decreased. Many interpersonal problems were raised which needed to be seen outside the context of stuttering. It is probable that there is a point in time when continuation of treatment is detrimental, actually encouraging the person to keep on seeing things in relation to the existence or non-existence of stuttering. The construct of stuttering could be kept alive rather than being allowed to die a natural death. It might well have been more beneficial to Luke if the treatment sessions had been tailed off earlier so as to enable him to experiment with new role relationships rather than with fluency itself. This is certainly my opinion now after the evidence that speech improvements continue to occur every sixteen weeks even when we might have only met twice during that time.

Whatever the final verdict, this form of treatment goes far beyond the reduction of the speech defect itself. It is seen as having to continue until the fluent person has sufficient ways of interpreting himself and others to make reasonably accurate predictions possible. What is "sufficient" is a matter of conjecture at this time, on which only further research can throw light.

After having finished reading all the transcripts, Dr. Bannister expressed his views on the psychotherapeutic approach and on how it differs from other psychotherapies as follows:

One very interesting feature of the whole psychotherapeutic method is that it seems to dispense with the use of "hydraulic" concepts for both therapist and patient. What I mean here is that the continual focus on the content and meaning of the stuttering situation and the fluent situation seems to rule out very effectively the use of vague notions such as "anxiety" and "depression". True, they appear from time to time, but you don't seem to get this focus you have with an enormous number of patients that they are the passive victims of internal forces which just gripped them so that they suffer "from depression" or are overcome by "anxiety" and so forth. It seems to force the patient into looking for meaning, looking for significance in his stuttering or not stuttering, so that he is never allowed to get away with the idea of a sort of "free floating stuttering".

Comparing it while I was reading it with other forms of psychotherapy, the big difference in practice, seems to be that somehow it either comprises the features of behaviour therapy and general psychotherapy or, to put it another way round, it is different from either. In particular, what I am thinking of, is the way the discussions always stay with the central topic of stammering, but yet go everywhere that can be traced out from the central topic, provided that there is some logical line of connection. Thus, on the one hand, it differs enormously from behaviour therapy in this fantastic degree of discussion, reconstruing, examination of the stuttering and fluent experience. On the other hand, it is quite unlike say personal construct theory psychotherapy *in general*, or client centred therapy or other types, in that the patient is never allowed to range away over life problems or to reformulate the entire nature of his complaint and so on and so forth. He is allowed to follow the line out from stuttering very extensively but it is a line *from stuttering* and returns to it and resettles as its focus on stuttering again every time.

Section V

The Future

CHAPTER 10

The Future

What we have said about the experience of the individual man holds true also for the scientist. A scientist formulates a theory—a body of constructs with a focus and a range of convenience. If he is a good scientist, he immediately starts putting it to test. It is almost certain that, as soon as he starts testing, he will also have to start changing it in the light of the outcomes. Any theory, then, tends to be transient. And the more practical it is and the more useful it appears to be, the more vulnerable it is to new evidence. Our own theory, particularly if it proves to be practical, will also have to be considered expendable in the light of tomorrow's outlooks and discoveries. At best it is an *ad interim* theory.

Kelly (1955)

I. Some Questions Answered

In actual fact, there was really only one central question that was asked by this research: is there a relationship between the way a stutterer sees himself and his world and variation in the severity of his stuttering? The simple answer is "yes, there is"; a relationship was found. These stutterers, as a group, developed increasingly elaborated systems of meaning concerning themselves as fluent speakers.

That there should have been a highly negative relationship between the view of "fluent self" and "stuttering self" (as one became more meaningful the other became less so) was not predicted. The theory was not sufficiently elaborated at the start of the research for such an event to be predicted. However, that this could have been done is suggested by the fact that one of the more implicit questions received a positive answer. This concerned the range of convenience of personal construct theory. So many theories disappoint because they become over-stretched when their exponents attempt to make them account for phenomena outside their original focus of convenience. But the reported research demonstrates that construct theory can account for a human phenomenon such as stuttering, suggesting that the range of convenience of the theory has not yet been tested to its limits. This being so, then the "way of life" theory of stuttering could itself have been extended to predict that, as one construct sub-system is elaborated the other, opposing one, is constricted.

229

In retrospect, it was probably a modicum of scepticism that prevented this theory of stuttering being expanded further. There was a philosophy of "well, let's see if the theory can get this far before spending more time on what may be a pointless task". Now it seems that it was not a pointless task and that further elaborations could be worth while.

Another implicit question that seems to have been answered concerns the nature of stuttering itself. There was certainly room for doubt as to whether stuttering severity could be reduced without manipulating the speech defect itself. It would be fair to say that the vast majority of treatment procedures include *some* focusing on what the stutterer actually does during speech. With some approaches he is only given "speech aids" to use whenever he finds himself "stuck", while with others the main emphasis is on the speech performance, and "attitudes" are considered of secondary importance. In this treatment it can definitely be stated that at no time was there any attempt to help the stutterer by giving him "speech aids" of any sort. As the severity of stuttering was reduced, there sometimes came a time when the occasions on which the person had trouble were analysed, and this might include minute discussions of specific troublesome letters, but this always took place within the context of the *meaning* of these letters or occasions for the individual. Whether such a rigorous adherence to the psychological rather than the behavioural aspects of stuttering is most advantageous for all stutterers is an, as yet, unanswered question.

II. Some Questions Raised

In the latter years of his thinking, Kelly became more and more convinced that it was useful to consider that behaviour was a way of asking questions.

> Instead of being a problem of threatening proportions, requiring the utmost explanation and control to keep man out of trouble, behaviour presents itself as man's principal instrument of inquiry. Without it his questions are academic and he gets nowhere. When it is prescribed for him he runs around in dogmatic circles. But when he uses it boldly to ask questions, a flood of unexpected answers rises to tax his utmost capacity to understand.
>
> It is true that in most psychology's inquiries some patently desirable behaviour is sought as an answer to the questions posed. But the quest always proves to be elusive. In the restless and wonderful world of humanistic endeavour, behaviour, however it may once have been intended as the embodiment of a conclusive answer, inevitably transforms itself into a further question—a question so compellingly posed by its enactment that, willy nilly, the actor finds that he has launched another experiment. Behaviour is indeed a question posed in such a way as to commit man to the role and obligation of an experiment. (Kelly, 1970, p. 260.)

What questions the stutterer is posing by his form of communication have still to be thought out. But one approach to the stuttering child might be to explore with him the answers he is seeking by his stumbling attempts to communicate. Here is another assumption of course; perhaps one of the questions he is asking is what the answer is if he *fails* to communicate. However, all these scientific hypotheses must wait for more research to suggest some of the answers.

Type of Therapy

While this research quest provided one or two answers, it raised many more questions. One concerns the therapeutic approach. Kelly approached people and their problems within the framework of his own personal construct system. In doing so he suggested one form of treatment which he found useful with some people and which best demonstrated the application of personal construct theory—this was Fixed Role Therapy. But this is not necessarily the best for all therapists nor for all clients. It was not considered to be the most appropriate in this instance. The particular approach to stutterers reported here is demonstrated in the chapter on therapy, which gives extensive excerpts from the tape recorded interviews with one stutterer. But there is no reason to suppose that this is the most appropriate for all those who might want to put this theoretical approach into practice.

It is probably true to say that if one observed a dozen people who say they are doing "personal construct theory psychotherapy", they will seem to have very little in common. However, they have, in fact, a great deal in common. They are all interpreting the situations in construct theory terms; are all using such Kellian notions as anxiety and hostility; are all thinking of construing systems in terms of tightening and loosening and so forth. The method is personal, the framework general. Bannister and Fransella sum the position up as follows:

> Looked at from the standpoint of personal construct theory, many current "psychotherapies" are better viewed as isolated *techniques* rather than as total approaches in their own right. Thus a construct theory psychotherapy might well include behaviour therapy methods, if the patient was having difficulty in tightening his construing in a given area. It might include a psychoanalytic type of free association if the patient had difficulty in loosening his constructs. But the construct theory psychotherapist would retain throughout the view that the client is essentially an experimental scientist in his own right, rather than someone to be manipulated by the behaviour therapist or absolved by the analyst. (Bannister and Fransella, 1971, p. 132.)

Although it was mandatory that no mechanical speech aids should be used in this research project, there is no reason why they should not be considered in the everyday therapy situation. One of the questions raised by this research is how best to deal with the very severe stutterer and the one of low intelligence. The treatment, in its research form, failed dismally to help these two. Indeed, mechanical devices may be essential with the very severe stutterer. In the research sample there was the young man whose speech was so severely disrupted that communication was almost impossible. The construct theory approach was impotent in the face of such a person, concentrating as it does on the experiencing and construing of fluency. Some mechanical control of the speech would now be considered an essential first step in such a case. But there is no need to limit oneself just to mechanical devices, such as rhythmically controlled speech. Any method that enables the stutterer to experience the speaking situation in a way different from that to which he is used, may be a help toward psychological reconstruction.

The same principle applies for the stutterer of low intelligence. It may be easier for him to elaborate his construing of himself as a nonstutterer by being able to speak for a time with rhythmic or syllabic speech. Subsequent experience has shown that it can be useful for the not so intelligent stutterer to analyse those situations in which he (as a stutterer) is traditionally fluent. For instance, with dogs and children. Why, *for him*, is this so? What are the factors in these situations which enable him to be fluent? A knowledge of some of these answers then allows one to help him apply the constructions to other situations in which he stutters and so, hopefully, to reconstrue them.

However, when one uses mechanical aids it is important, from a theoretical standpoint, that the person does not come to regard them as an end in themselves. The stutterer will only be able to generalize from these artificial speech situations if he can be helped to construe the different reactions he gets and the different feelings he has. He should be encouraged to use at least some of the same construct dimensions to construe reactions to his "artificial speech" that he will come to use to construe reactions to his future fluent speech.

The Therapeutic Process

Apart from the form of the therapeutic programme, innumerable questions have been raised about the nature of the therapeutic process itself. By and large, all these questions relate to personal construct theory and the nature of psychological change rather than being specific to this present study. There are three main questions to which answers might be sought. The first concerns prognosis. How can one gather reliable information from the stutterer which will enable one to predict whether he is likely to improve or not? Of course, ideally speaking, everyone should improve. It is the idiocy of the therapist in not being able to see exactly how to help the person bring about his psychological change that is to blame. But within the limits of one's capabilities it is essential to strive to produce methods for predicting likelihood of improvement.

There have been vague suggestions in this study about where it might be profitable to look for answers. The most promising seems to be the finding that there is a difference between those who improved and those who did not improve (coupled with those who opted out of treatment prematurely) on the grid saturation score. The more highly organized the system, the less likelihood there was of improvement, and the more likelihood there was that the stutterer would leave treatment before the therapist thought he should. Not only might this be developed as a guide as to whether a stutterer is likely to benefit from treatment, but also as an indicator of whether treatment should be terminated because of premature tightening of construing. This latter information could also be of importance if the treatment is going to continue, since it would indicate the need for different strategies to be adopted.

The notion of a measure of construct permeability (or whatever its final theoretical status turns out to be) is also an area of research concerning the basic therapeutic process itself. How can one monitor such changes and so predict consequences such as anxiety, hostility or aggression and so forth? What other operational definitions of theoretical constructs can be developed? Grid technique at the present time is a laborious process. Perhaps in time the person will be able to feed his grid or other responses directly into a computer. This will result in overcoming one of the main hurdles in the use of grids in the therapeutic situation. The person has probably psychologically moved a long way from the point at which he completed the grid by the time the therapist receives the grid results. What is needed is some on-line computer system which will give an indication of the present state of a particular aspect of a person's construing system at a particular point in time.

Duration of Therapy

Another question raised by this research is whether it is necessary to take so long in bringing about improvement. One of the arguments for the treatment being prolonged is that learning to live the life of the fluent speaker can only be begun when there is a considerable amount of consistent fluency. Further work with stutterers has continued to justify the importance placed on this extra time spent. An attempt at speeding up the recovery process met with considerable success in the first place, but the relapse rate shot up. There is probably a very delicate balance to be drawn here between the desire to discharge a person when he has reached a satisfactory level of fluency and the stability of his "new" way of seeing life. The questions of the nature of this balance and what is actually meant by "stability" have still to be answered. One question that has also to be clarified is whether there is an optimum rate at which psychological change occurs for each individual. Certainly, Luke seemed only to conduct fluency experiments at "new" levels of fluency once every fifteen or sixteen weeks. If there is some such process operating for all individuals, although not necessarily at such long intervals, then follow-up sessions for those who have treatment on an intensive basis over a relatively short period of time would seem essential.

The "Way of Life" Theory's Range of Convenience

The last question to be discussed concerns the range of convenience of the theory put forward to account for stuttering behaviour. The question is really two-fold. First, can it account for changes in stuttering severity resulting from other forms of treatment? Second, can it provide an explanation of the maintenance of other long-standing behavioural disorders?

A Common Denominator in Treatments of Stuttering. If there is some support for the hypothesis that an *increase in meaningfulness of being a fluent speaker is related to a decrease in the severity of stuttering*, then it could be considered as a common factor running through *all* instances in which a person has moved successfully from stuttering to fluency. This is not meant to imply that the form the therapy takes is irrelevant, but rather that a successful outcome results from treatment that has enabled the individual to reconstrue situations from the point of view of a fluent speaker which he had previously construed from the standpoint of a stutterer. Operant techniques are right for some, while group therapy is best for others.

A pilot study has been conducted, more in hope than expectancy, with a sample of eleven stutterers tested at the beginning and end of treatment and having different forms of treatment. The inadequacy of this sample was determined at the outset by the fact that nine of the eleven stutterers had the same type of treatment. This was an intensive group procedure, four weeks in duration and four hours a day. During this time, syllable speech and block modification techniques were used together with situation assignments designed to bring about attitude change. Of the remaining two stutterers in the sample, one received syllabic speech coupled with psychotherapy and the other a form of desensitization.

Apart from the bias in favour of one particular form of treatment, two other problems arose. The first was that most of the stutterers tested after having eighty hours of syllabic speech found it extremely difficult, if not impossible, to speak without breaking their words up into syllables in a test situation. The speech measures thus obtained were not a valid representation of their actual level of speech fluency. In future, it will be arranged that the post-treatment testing will take place some two or three weeks after the end of the course when it is hoped that the stutterers will have overcome their difficulty in speaking "naturally".

A second obstacle that rapidly became apparent was the time-consuming nature of the administration of a bi-polar implications grid. With a maximum of one hour available for testing, the use of these grids was a practical impossibility. Hinkle's original form was therefore used with four instead of six photographs for the elicitation of constructs. In Hinkle's method, the two poles of a pair of constructs are compared and the person is asked to consider whether switching from one pole to the other on a construct will involve similar switches on others. All constructs are paired in this way and the Impgrid built up from these implied linkages.

With this control group of eleven stutterers, there were found to be no significant relationships between the speech measures and change in the number of construct implications, although all changes were in the predicted direction. In fact, small sample size and the use of syllabic speech during final testing militated against the finding of differences at a significant level. As for speech improvement, these stutterers had a reduction of 26·3% in disfluent words and 11·4% in total disfluencies, the two measures correlating 0·91. Taking the criterion of improvement of 50% reduction in disfluencies, then four or 36·4% improved, three became worse on the total disfluency measure and two worse on the disfluent word count. No follow-up was carried out. It could be argued that the act of trying *not* to use syllabic speech during testing had an adverse effect on fluency, but there was no evidence of this.

There is no evidence, in fact, that treating stutterers in groups is any more successful than that achieved on an individual basis. There is no evidence as to the effectiveness of group procedures at all if it comes to that. The group method is obviously of advantage to therapists when people are waiting impatiently on the doorstep for treatment. But from the construct theory standpoint one wonders whether intensive programmes covering a relatively short period of time could be expected to be very successful for the majority. If stuttering is indeed a way of life, then there can be few who are able to change their way of life in so short a space of time. It is only when fluency, however limited in amount, is available to the stutterer that he can begin to reconstrue. The use of syllabic speech can be a great help in enabling the stutterer to experiment in situations normally withheld from him, providing he construes along some of the dimensions he uses for his fluent speech. The assumption cannot be made that placing the stutterer in a "situation" will automatically enable him to reconstrue it and that such construing will automatically be beneficial. Maybe he will not like some of the answers he gets to his speaking experiments. Even if he does approve of the results, how easily will he be able to generalize these to other situations without help?

Perhaps a construct theory approach to group psychotherapy might provide more guide-lines. It might start off by finding out, for each individual, his or her particular stuttering-provoking situations using the "situations grid". Future assignments could then be geared for the individual within a group context. Kelly outlined six phases in a group therapeutic procedure designed to bring about reconstruction. First of all, the individuals have to feel they have the support of at least some of the other members of the group. This support or acceptance is defined as the perception that others are ready "to see the world through another person's eyes". Kelly suggested the use of role playing here, but other ways can be devised to bring about the same result.

This feeling of acceptance allows the second stage of *initiation of primary role relationships* to proceed. It is this particular stage that Kelly thought gave group therapy its advantage over individual therapy. When some piece of role playing has taken place between two or three members, the non-participants are asked to say what the role players may have felt at certain stages of the enactment. They are being asked to subsume the others' constructs and so play a role in relation to them. The role players tell the non-participants how accurate their interpretations were and so give immediate validation of the non-participants role construing. Use could be made here of the stuttering-provoking hierarchies. "Difficult" roles could be played (difficult for the individual that is) and then followed by a discussion as to why Mr. X found them "difficult" and so forth. The roles must be carefully allotted and it is the interpretation of the roles by the others that shows the group members alternative ways of construing situations or people with which they have difficulty. Just as it is hypothesized that there is a common denominator in successful treatments of stuttering, so there is a common denominator running through group members' role enactments—improvement occurs from those which give the person an alternative view to an old construction.

The third stage of *initiation of mutual primary enterprises* involves the group in designing their own enactments and experiments based on their understanding of each other. All experimenting is done inside the group at this stage, within one group session. The next stage of *exploration of personal problems* can now take place because the members should feel well supported and understood by the others and so minimizing threat.

At the fifth stage, the members *explore secondary roles*, they enact situations related to outside events and outside persons and then at stage six, they *explore secondary enterprises* by experimenting with the new roles outside the group.

This systematic use of the group to enable new role relationships to be developed within the framework of fluency has not yet been put into practice in the treatment of stutterers. But, just as with construct theory therapy for the individual, the advantages of carrying out treatment within a highly explicit theoretical framework along with methods of measurement will help define the parameters of the improvement process and causes of success and failure.

A Common Denominator in Long-Standing Behavioural Complaints. Stuttering has been seen in terms of meaning of the behaviour. It is more meaningful in verbal interactions to be a stutterer (for a stutterer) than to be a fluent speaker. This does not mean that he *wants* to speak like he does, indeed most would dearly like to be fluent. But if our way of behaving is governed by our way of construing then we cannot just volunteer to step off into a largely poorly construed world.

The dimensions along which we construe ourselves and others may well be important determinants of our behaviour. Take the over-weight woman. Over-weight clearly has meaning for her. People relate to her as *a fat person*. She is subsumed under such stereotypes as "a fat person is a jolly person". Supposing she were suddenly to lose weight and become around average, surely she would need to develop a very different conception of herself. If she is young, she might find out that young men find her attractive and make advances to her, whereas before they had remained companions. She could well be expected to experience anxiety at this turn of events because *the events with which she was confronted lie outside the range of convenience of her construct system*. She does not know how to react to this ardent young man and he, in turn, may misconstrue her diffident behaviour. The theory of stuttering could be applied to this obese woman. No permanent weight loss will be achieved until *the meaning of being a woman of normal weight is at least as meaningful to her as being a fat woman*. Two studies using repertory grid technique have so far shown how changes in the construing of the self have accompanied weight change (Fransella, 1970c; Fransella and Crisp, 1970). They march hand in hand, or perhaps more accurately one behind the other. The evidence suggests that changes in the view of the self may precede relapse but this finding has yet to be replicated.

Take the agoraphobic as another example. Here is someone who has centred his, or more probably her, life around not going out of doors. This way of life is meaningful—being someone who can take or leave the wide open spaces is not. Psychotherapy for such complaints often focuses on seeking to identify the "meaning" of the fear of the out-doors for the patient. Behaviour therapy focuses on enabling the patient to reconstrue the out-door situations as an end in themselves. But what is often not reported in any detail is the time spent in discussion of the patient's "problems". This means a discussion of the significance of being able to go out and about. It is not intended to imply that such procedures are ineffective and that the one advocated here *is* effective. But it is suggested that it may be *more* effective to incorporate a number of behavioural complaints under one theoretical umbrella than dealing with each piece of "behaviour" under one heading and "attitudes" under another.

This theoretical approach could equally well be applied to the smoker who may construe smoking as a sign of maturity, social sophistication or a screen behind which to hide; also to the ticqueur or the lisper or the hypochondriac—all of whom have learnt to construe their world in relation to themselves as ticqueur, lisper or hypochondriac. Obesity has meaning for the obese, smoking for the smoker, lisping for the lisper and stuttering for the stutterer.

One final example of the application of the "way of life" theory beyond its focus of convenience—stuttering—concerns the obsessional neurotic. It has been suggested (Fransella, 1972) that the obsessional has so restricted his way of life that the only area of meaning remaining to him is that centred around his obsessions. Therapy is thus seen as aiming to help him to increase the range of convenience of his construct system so that he can deal with an increasing rather than a decreasing number of events.

III. Conclusion

All the examples given to illustrate the potential range of convenience of the theory proposed are speculative and so go far beyond the existing evidence. However, one of the functions of psychological research is to enable the scientist to start looking at the next step leading toward the greater understanding of the human predicament. Kelly stressed the notion of *man-the-scientist*—someone whose aim is to predict and control events in his environment. Stutterers, ticqueurs, smokers, obsessionals, the obese and others remain as they are because they function best as scientists in this way. They need help in devising theories which will produce sufficient validating evidence to enable them to establish themselves in their own idiosyncratic way as non-stutterers, non-ticqueurs, or non-smokers and so forth.

Appendix 1

THE STATISTICAL ANALYSIS OF THE BI-POLAR IMPGRID

The purpose of this analysis is to calculate the probability of a relationship between any two concepts included in a bi-polar implications grid. Let lines X and Y in Fig. 23 represent any two lines of such a grid, line X gives the subject's

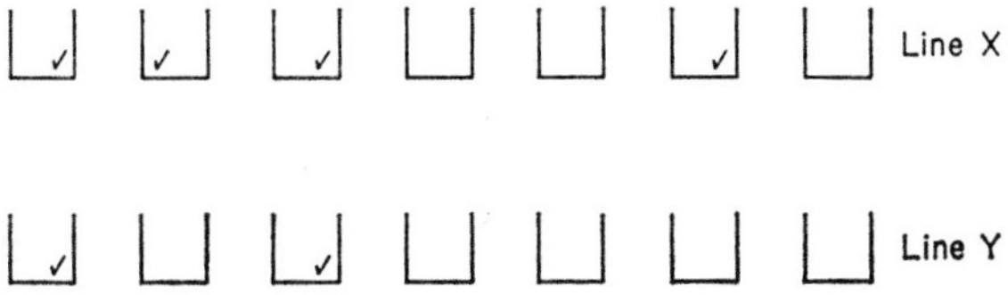

FIG. 23 Two lines of an implications grid (bi-polar) with implications represented by a tick.

response to one concept; line Y his response to another. In each line there are seven boxes, with the possibility of only one tick per box. The probability of a tick in any box will vary from line to line, that is from concept to concept; depending on the subject's response to that concept.

In line X there are four ticks in seven boxes, hence the probability of a ticked box, assuming all boxes are equally likely to be ticked, is $px = 4/7$. The probability of a non-ticked (blank) box is given by $qx = (1 - px) = 3/7$.

Similarly for line Y. Where there is a total of two ticks, the probability of a ticked box is $py = 2/7$, and the probability of a blank box is $qy = (1 - py) = 5/7$.

In calculating the probability of the relation between any two lines occurring by chance, it is necessary to consider the nine different ways in which a box in one line can be related to the corresponding box in another line.

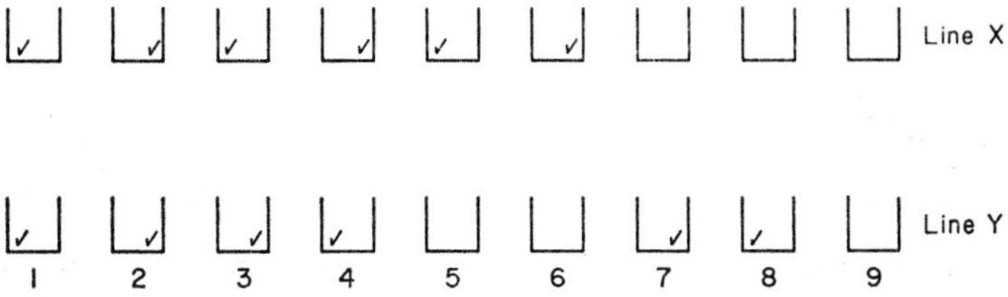

FIG. 24 Nine ways in which implications can be related in a bi-polar implications grid.

Figure 24 shows these nine possible relationships. The first boxes of lines X and Y in Fig. 23 are an example of a "type 2" relationship, whereas the last boxes are an example of a "type 9" relationship,

The probability of types 1 or 2 or 3 or 4 is $= px \cdot py$

i.e. the probability of a ticked box in line X times the probability of a ticked box in line Y.

239

The probability of types 5 or 6 $= px.qy$

i.e. the probability of a ticked box in line X times the probability of an unticked box in line Y.

The probability of types 7 or 8 $= qx.py$

i.e. the probability of an unticked box in line X times the probability of a ticked box in line Y.

The probability of type 9 $= qx.qy$

i.e. the probability of an unticked box in line X times the probability of an unticked box in line Y.

Hence

$$P_1 = \frac{px.py}{4}$$

$$P_2 = \frac{px.py}{4}$$

$$P_3 = \frac{px.py}{4}$$

$$P_4 = \frac{px.py}{4}$$

$$P_5 = \frac{px.qy}{2}$$

$$P_6 = \frac{px.pq}{2}$$

$$P_7 = \frac{qx.py}{2}$$

$$P_8 = \frac{qx.py}{2}$$

$$P_9 = qx.qy$$

The probability of the relationship between any two lines occurring by chance, is the product of the probabilities of the relationship between the individual boxes.

In analysing this test, positive or negative implications only are considered. By positive implications is meant those of type 1 or type 2; by negative implications is meant those of type 3 or type 4. The probability of positive implications is given by $p_+ = p_1 + p_2 = \dfrac{px.py}{2}$

Hence $q_+ = \dfrac{(1 - px.py)}{2}$

Similarly the probability of a negative implication is given by

$$p_- = p_3 + p_4 = \frac{px.py}{2} \quad \text{and} \quad q_- = \frac{(1 - px.py)}{2}$$

In Fig. 24, there are two boxes (1 and 2) with positive implications, the probability of this occurring by chance is $p = {}^nC_r p_+{}^r . q_+{}^{n-r}$ (where n = number of boxes per line; r = number of positive implications) $= {}^7C_2 \dfrac{(px.py)^2}{2} \dfrac{(1 - px.py)^5}{2}$

There are no boxes with negative implications hence the probability of this occurring by chance is $p = {}^nC_r p_-{}^r q_-{}^{n-r} = \dfrac{(1 - px.py)^7}{2}$

If the probability of positive implications, or negative implications falls below the chosen level of significance then the null hypothesis that the apparent relation between the two lines is due to chance may be rejected.

This test is two-tailed, that is to say, there may be a significant absence of, say, negative implications, as well as a significant number of positive implications between two lines.

Appendix 2

1. *Social interaction:*
Any statement in which face-to-face, on-going, continuing interaction or lack of face-to-face, on-going, continuing interaction with others is clearly indicated.

Interjudge reliability

(a) active 75%
(b) inactive 75%

Rating Category	Number of Stutterers	Grids		Constructs		Opposite Pole
		S.	NS.	Super-ordinate	Sub-ordinate	
Aggravating	3	2	1	1	2	Crawlers and snides
Outspoken	3	1	2	0	3	Not able to bring pressure to bear on people
Persuasive	3	Both		2	1	
Lonely	4	0	4	4	0	Have friends
Isolated	9	Both		9	0	Do not get ostracised
Desire privacy	1	0	1	1	0	
Hurtful	3	1	2	1	2	Do not take the mickey out of others
Shy/reserved	17	Both		Both		
Desire to please	2	1	1	0	2	
Friendly	14	Both		Both		
Good conversationalists	9	Both		Both		Stand back and listen
Mix well	17	Both		Both		
Liked	8	Both		Both		
Interesting	9	3	6	5	4	Short of words
Talkative	8	Both		0	8	Outspoken
Wary	5	2	3	2	3	
Boring	7	Both		Both		
Homely	7	Both		1	6	Not easy to live with
Listeners/Observers	5	5	1	3	2	Sly
Open	8	Both		Both		
Ill-mannered	2	0	2	0	2	
Laughed at	2	2	0	1	1	
Stand out in a group	6	6	0	Both		Nondescript

2. Forcefulness:

Any statement denoting energy, over expressiveness, persistence, intensity, or the opposite.

Interjudge reliability
(a) High 75%
(b) Low 75%

Rating Category	Number of Stutterers	Grids S.	Grids NS.	Constructs Super-ordinate	Constructs sub-ordinate	Opposite Pole
Domineering	10	Mainly non-stutt.		Both		Do not Fight back
Creative	1	0	1	0	1	
Independent	10	2	8	7	3	Need others
Argumentative	1	0	1	1	0	
Weak	8	Both		Both		Strong minded
Sarcastic	1	Both		0	1	
Impulsive	1	Both		1	0	
Aware	3	Both		Both		Have little idea of what's going on
Get something out of life	5	Both		5	0	
Lazy	6	Both		3	3	
Active	3	Both		1	2	
Relaxed	14	Both		Both		Sloppy
Serious	13	Both		Both		

3. Organization:

Any statement denoting either the state of or process of structuring, planning, and organizing, or the opposite. The statement should indicate that a person either has or lacks a general trait of structuring, organizing and planning ability or can be described as organized, structured or disorganized and unstructured.

Interjudge reliability
(a) High 75%
(b) Low 75%

Rating Category	Number of Stutterers	Grids S.	Grids NS.	Constructs Super-ordinate	Constructs sub-ordinate	Opposite Pole
Conventional	6	2	4	Both		
Efficient	5	Both		Both		
Able to plan ahead	2	1	1	2	1	
Logical	1	1	0	1	0	

4. Self-sufficiency:

Any statement denoting independence, initiative, confidence and ability to solve one's own problems, or the opposite.

Interjudge reliability
(a) High 65%
(b) Low 65%

Item					Opposite
Confident	11	1	1	1	
Mature	4	Both	Both	1	
Secure	2	1	3	0	
Unable to cope	4	4	Both	0	
Feel inferior	2	Both	2	0	

5. Status:

Any statement wherein references are made to either status or to high prestige status symbols, or to a lack of status striving or to low prestige status symbols.

Interjudge reliability
(a) High 75%
(b) Low 75%

Item					Opposite
Ambitious	12	1	Both	8	4	Not cool and calculating
Successful	5	1	4	4	1	Not likely to make their mark in the world
Sophisticated	3	0	3	0	3	Ordinary
Get good jobs	2	2	0	1	1	Social inferiors
Upper class	3	1	2	0	3	Muddle through life
Get things done	4	3	1	3	0	
Initiative	3	1	2	3	0	
Achieve their aims	1	0	1	1	0	
Respected	9	Both		7	2	Despised by others
Educated	12	4	8	3	9	Technical types
Have money	1	1	0	0	1	
Superior	2	0	2	2	0	Do not matter

6. Factual description:

A characteristic so described that most observers could agree to the description as something factual. A fact would be a characteristic not open to question.

Interjudge reliability
(a) Not known
(b) Not known

Item					Opposite
Young	4	3	1	0	4	
Married	1	1	0	0	1	
Office workers	5	1	4	0	5	Not managerial types

Rating Category	Number of Stutterers	Grids		Constructs		Opposite Pole
		S.	NS.	Super-ordinate	Sub-ordinate	
7. Intellective:						
Knowledgeable	13	Both		8	5	Bluff their way through life
Intelligent	13	Both		1	Both	Slow in the uptake
Fool	11	2	9		10	Do not think stutterers are fools

7. *Intellective:*
Any statement denoting intelligence or intellectual pursuits, or the opposite.

Interjudge reliability
(a) High   75%
(b) Low   75%

8. *Self-reference:*
Any statement in which the person taking the test refers directly to himself.
This was not used since the design of the elicitation procedure makes it highly likely that the majority of constructs will be self reference.

Rating Category	Number of Stutterers	Grids		Constructs		Opposite Pole
		S.	NS.	Super-ordinate	Sub-ordinate	
9. Imagination						
Dreamers	4	1	3	4	0	Realist

9. *Imagination*
Any statement denoting activity which is supplemental to or divorced from reality, or its opposite.
Interjudge reliability
(a) Not known
(b) Low 75%

10. Alternatives:

(a) The subject employs more than one description, (b) employs qualified description suggesting the possibility of other descriptions, (c) used descriptions suggesting a strong openness or (d) closeness to new alternatives.
Interjudge reliability
(a) 59%

Broadminded	6	Both	6	0	Dogmatic
Sensitive	8	Both	Both		

11. Sexual:

Any direct reference to sexual behaviour or implicit sexual behaviour, positive or negative.
Interjudge reliability
(a) 59%

Attractive	4	0	4	2	2

12. Morality:

Any statement denoting religious or moral values.
Interjudge reliability
(a) High 75%
(b) Low 65%

Religious	2	Both		1	
Honest	9	Both	Both		1
Truthful	2	0	2		
Conscientious	8	Both	2	Both	0 — Do not wonder what is right or wrong
Reliable	5	1	4	4	1

13. External Appearance:

Any statement describing a person's appearance which may be either more objective or more subjective.
Interjudge reliability
(a) Not known
(b) Not known

Scruffy	1	1	0	1	Good looking
Masculine	1	0	1	0	1
Feminine	1	0	1	1	0
Well-groomed	5	3	2	1	4

		Grids		Constructs		
Rating Category	Number of Stutterers	S.	NS.	Super-ordinate	Sub-ordinate	Opposite Pole
14. *Emotional arousal:* Any statement denoting a transient or chronic readiness to react with stronger feelings such as anger, anxiety, disgust, enthusiasm, fearfulness, grief, joy, nervousness, surprise, yearning etc.						
Worry	8		Both	4	4	Have peace of mind
Irritable	7	5	2	5	2	Unruffled
Tense	5	5	0	0	5	
Ruled by emotions	2	1	1	2	0	
Intolerant/ impatient	6	5	1	5	1	Suffer fools gladly
Uncompromizing	2	1	1	2	0	Moan if anything goes wrong
Interjudge reliability (a) 75%						
Depressed	1	0	1	1	0	
Happy	14	Both		12	2	
Controlled	2	Both		1	1	Easily embarrassed
15. *Diffuse generalization:* Undifferentiated statements which are applicable to almost anyone, such as non-specific personal judgements, or social clichés. They often are not scorable able in other categories because of their generality or great ambiguity. Interjudge reliability (a) Not known (b) Not known						
Good personality	3	1	2	1	2	
Normal	4	3	1	0	4	
Complete people	1	0	1	1	0	
Stand out in a crowd	6	6	0	Both		Nondescript

16. Egoism:

Any statement denoting self-importance or a lack of self-importance. High egoism may be either constructive or destructive and will be more literal— not debating whether, for example, the conceited person really is confident.

Word						
Noticed by people	2	1	1	1	1	
Smug	4	Both				Not pleased with themselves
Self confident	9	Both				
Over confident	4	1	3	0	4	
Selfish	10	Both				
Snob	5	4	1	3	1	Do not ride rough shod over people

Interjudge reliability
(a) High   75%
(b) Low   not known

17. Tenderness:

Any statement denoting susceptibility to softer feelings toward others such as love, compassion, gentleness, kindness, considerateness, or the opposite.

Word					
Encouraging	3	3	0	1	
Sympathetic	13	Both			
Helpful	7	Both			
Discerning	5	1	4	2	Do not "see through" stutterers

Interjudge reliability
(a) High   75%
(b) Low   75%

18. Time orientation:

Any statement denoting a state of mind which strongly implies an individual's future orientation and expectancy, a part orientation and expectancy, or a present orientation and expectancy. Some descriptions may imply all three orientations and cannot be scored.

Word						
Believe in progress and change	4	1	3	3	1	
Pessimistic	4	1	3	4	0	Mistrust progress
Modern	5	Both		1	4	Frumpish

Interjudge reliability
(a) Past   75%
(b) Future   75%
(c) Present   59%

Rating Category	Number of Stutterers	Grids S.	Grids NS.	Constructs Super-ordinate	Constructs Sub-ordinate	Opposite Pole
Have responsibility	2	1	1	2	0	
Have interests	10	Both		8	2	Have a limited existence
Happy-go-lucky	11	Both		Both		
Thoughtful	4	1	3	4	0	Shallow

19. *Involvement:*

Any statement denoting a persistent working toward that which an individual finds more generally and internally meaningful or, restated, a high or low internal and more total commitment or dedication to and strong pursuit of an interest, occupation, way of life, philosophy, or simply the state of commitment, dedication or lack of such.

Interjudge reliability

(a) High   65%

(b) Low   75%

20. *Comparatives:*

Any description which uses the comparative form, i.e. relativity is introduced into the description which excluded a definite position, amount or quality.

This category was not used because of the very large number of comparative statements made.

21. Qualifiers:

Any adjective, adverb or phrase which makes a description extreme or suggests a high degree of the characteristics.

This category was not used because of the very large number of qualified statements made.

22. Humour:

Any statement specifically denoting either the ability or inability to perceive, appreciate, or express that which is funny, amusing or ludicrous.

Interjudge reliability

(a) High   75%
(b) Low   75%

Sense of humour	10	Both	2	8

Appendix 3

Analysis of construct implications for *self-non-self* and *stutterer-non-stutterer* that were used by ten or more stutterers and grouped under Landfield's construct content categories. "Consistent" responses are those shown in bold type.

SOCIAL INTERACTION

	Mix well		Not mix well		Nil response
	Self	Non-self	Self	Non-self	
Mix well					
Stutterers	**1**	0	0	0	1
Non-stutterers	0	**2**	1	0	7
Not mix well					
Stutterers	1	1	**3**	0	1
Non-stutterers	0	0	0	**0**	1
Nil response	5	2	2	3	3

SENSE OF HUMOUR

	Sense of Humour		Not Sense of Humour		Nil response
	Self	Non-self	Self	Non-self	
Sense of Humour					
Stutterers	**1**	0	0	0	0
Nonstutterers	0	**0**	0	0	0
Not Sense of Humour					
Stutterers	1	0	**0**	0	1
Nonstutterers	0	0	0	**0**	0
Nil response	6	0	0	7	4

TENDERNESS

	Sympathetic		Not sympathetic		Nil response
	Self	Non-self	Self	Non-self	
Sympathetic					
Stutterers	4	0	0	0	0
Nonstutterers	0	0	0	0	0
Not sympathetic					
Stutterers	1	0	0	0	0
Nonstutterers	0	0	0	3	0
Nil response	6	1	0	8	3

EGOISM

	Selfish		Not selfish		Nil response
	Self	Non-self	Self	Non-self	
Selfish					
Stutterers	0	0	3	0	0
Nonstutterers	0	0	0	0	0
Not selfish					
Stutterers	0	0	3	0	0
Nonstutterers	0	0	0	0	0
Nil response	0	6	2	0	6

FORCEFULNESS

	Relaxed		Not relaxed		Nil response
	Self	Non-self	Self	Non-self	
Relaxed					
Stutterers	**0**	0	1	0	1
Nonstutterers	0	**2**	0	1	1
Not relaxed					
Stutterers	3	0	**4**	0	0
Nonstutterers	0	0	0	**0**	0
Nil response	0	0	0	1	13

	Serious		Not serious		Nil response
	Self	Non-self	Self	Non-self	
Serious					
Stutterers	**3**	0	0	0	0
Nonstutterers	0	**0**	0	0	0
Not serious					
Stutterers	0	0	**0**	0	0
Nonstutterers	0	0	0	**1**	2
Nil response	2	3	4	4	7

SOCIAL INTERACTION

	Shy/Reserved		Not shy/Reserved		Nil response
	Self	Non-self	Self	Non-self	
Shy/Reserved					
Stutterers	6	0	1	0	1
Nonstutterers	0	0	0	0	0
Not shy/Reserved					
Stutterers	0	0	0	0	0
Nonstutterers	0	1	0	2	2
Nil response	2	0	3	4	10

	Friendly		Not friendly		Nil response
	Self	Non-self	Self	Non-self	
Friendly					
Stutterers	0	0	0	0	0
Nonstutterers	0	1	0	1	3
Not friendly					
Stutterers	2	0	0	0	3
Nonstutterers	0	0	0	0	0
Nil response	6	3	0	1	8

INTELLECTIVE

	Knowledgeable		Not knowledgeable		Nil response
	Self	Non-self	Self	Non-self	
Knowledgeable					
Stutterers	2	0	0	0	0
Nonstutterers	0	1	0	0	1
Not knowledgeable					
Stutterers	0	0	2	0	0
Nonstutterers	0	0	0	0	0
Nil response	6	1	0	4	9

	Intelligent		Not intelligent		Nil response
	Self	Non-self	Self	Non-self	
Intelligent					
Stutterers	2	0	0	0	1
Nonstutterers	0	0	0	1	0
Not intelligent					
Stutterers	0	0	0	0	0
Nonstutterers	0	0	0	0	0
Nil response	6	3	1	6	6

INVOLVEMENT

	Have interests		Not have interests		Nil response
	Self	Non-self	Self	Non-self	
Have interests					
Stutterers	1	0	0	0	0
Nonstutterers	0	0	0	0	1
Not have interests					
Stutterers	2	0	2	0	1
Nonstutterers	0	0	0	0	0
Nil response	1	2	1	2	7

	Happy-go-lucky		Not happy-go-lucky		Nil response
	Self	Non-self	Self	Non-self	
Happy-go-lucky					
Stutterers	0	0	0	0	0
Nonstutterers	0	0	0	1	1
Not happy-go-lucky					
Stutterers	1	0	1	0	0
Nonstutterers	0	0	0	0	0
Nil response	4	2	1	3	8

STATUS

	Ambitious		Not ambitious		Nil response
	Self	Non-self	Self	Non-self	
Ambitious					
Stutterers	**0**	0	0	0	0
Nonstutterers	1	**2**	0	1	0
Not ambitious					
Stutterers	2	0	**0**	0	1
Nonstutterers	0	0	0	**0**	0
Nil response	1	0	0	2	14

	Educated		Not educated		Nil response
	Self	Non-self	Self	Non-self	
Educated					
Stutterers	**2**	0	0	0	0
Nonstutterers	0	**0**	0	2	0
Not educated					
Stutterers	3	0	**0**	0	2
Nonstutterers	0	2	0	**0**	0
Nil response	4	0	0	4	5

FORCEFULNESS

| | Domineering | | Not domineering | | Nil response |
	Self	Non-self	Self	Non-self	
Domineering					
Stutterers	**1**	0	0	0	0
Nonstutterers	0	**1**	0	0	0
Not domineering					
Stutterers	0	0	**2**	0	1
Nonstutterers	0	0	0	**0**	0
Nil response	1	4	4	1	5

| | Independent | | Not independent | | Nil response |
	Self	Non-self	Self	Non-self	
Independent					
Stutterers	**0**	0	0	0	0
Nonstutterers	1	**0**	0	0	0
Not independent					
Stutterers	0	0	**0**	0	1
Nonstutterers	0	0	0	**0**	0
Nil response	5	1	0	4	8

EMOTIONAL AROUSAL

	Happy		Not happy		Nil response
	Self	Non-self	Self	Non-self	
Happy					
Stutterers	**0**	0	0	0	1
Nonstutterers	0	**3**	0	2	1
Not happy					
Stutterers	2	0	**4**	0	2
Nonstutterers	0	0	0	**0**	0
Nil response	1	1	0	3	8

SELF-SUFFICIENT

	Confident		Not confident		Nil response
	Self	Non-self	Self	Non-self	
Confident					
Stutterers	**0**	0	0	0	0
Nonstutterers	0	**4**	0	1	0
Not confident					
Stutterers	4	0	**2**	0	1
Nonstutterers	0	0	0	**0**	0
Nil response	0	0	3	1	6

Constructs in N.S.2 Grid

1a More suave
1b Less suave
2a Earnest
2b Relaxed
3a Worthy of respect
3b Common
4a Aggressive
4b Gentle
5a Intelligent
5b Ordinary
6a Depth of character
6b Accept others' points of view without evidence
7a Like me in character
7b Not like me in character
8a Respected and looked up to
8b Not necessarily respected
9a A person who matters
9b A person who doesn't matter
10a Less chance of enjoying life to the full
10b More chance of enjoying life to the full
11a Have status
11b Do not have status
12a Less likely to be refused
12b Likely to be refused
13a Does not know how to get a person to change his mind
13b Knows how to get a person to change his mind
14a Able to have a greater appreciation of things
14b Not able to have a greater appreciation of things
15a Stutterers
15b Not stutterers

Constructs in N.S.3 Grid

1a Weak, unsure
1b Strong, sure
2a Carefree
2b Sober
3a Intellectual, better class
3b Ordinary
4a Desire to get on well with people, have bonhomie
4b Do not care about others' feelings
5a Like me in character
5b Not like me in character

6a Care about criticism
6b Do not care about criticism
7a Do not *know* if liked or not
7b Know if liked or not
8a *Care* if liked or not
8b Do not *care* if liked or not
9a Likely to be liked
9b Less likely to be liked
10a Do not try to make others think they are superior
10b Try to make others think they are superior
11a Do not have to handle situation of being disliked
11b May have to handle situation of being disliked
12a Stutterers
12b Fluent person

CONSTRUCTS IN N.S.4 GRID

1a Aloof
1b Want to be liked
2a Self-sufficient
2b Eager to make friends
3a Sophisticated
3b Ordinary
4a Self-confident
4b Lack self-confidence, must be "one of the lads"
5a Sense of humour
5b Serious
6a Kind and sympathetic
6b Less kind and sympathetic
7a Enjoy intellectual experiences
7b Unable to appreciate intellectual experiences
8a Like me in character
8b Not like me in character
9a Likely to be respected and liked
9b Not likely to be respected and liked
10a Not aware of the rewards friendships have to offer
10b Believe that making friends is satisfying and socially desirable
11a Independent
11b Dependent
12a Enjoy the humorous situations in life
12b Do not enjoy the humorous situations in life
13a Believe that one should 'do unto others as you would have done unto you'
13b Do not believe that one should 'do unto others as you would have done unto you'
14a Stutterers
14b A physically and mentally fluent person

CONSTRUCTS IN N.S.5 GRID

1a Relaxed
1b Tense, serious, on edge, concerned to do everything right
2a Confident

2b Unsure
3a Refined
3b Less refined
4a Articulate
4b Less articulate
5a Have authority
5b Receive authority
6a Intelligent
6b Less intelligent
7a Like me in character
7b Not like me in character
8a Enjoy life
8b Find life a strain
9a Interesting to talk to
9b Waste time making sure they are right
10a Respected
10b Not respected
11a Assert more influence on interpersonal relations
11b Do not assert much influence on interpersonal relations
12a Believe that interpersonal relations are of fundamental importance to one's life
12b Do not hold this belief
13a Communicate well
13b Communicate less well
14a Able to bring pressure to bear on people, making them more willing to agree with one
14b Not able to bring pressure to bear on people
15a Understand more things
15b Understand fewer things
16a Have basic feelings of inferiority
16b Do not have basic feelings of inferiority
17a Stutterers
17b Fluent speaker

Constructs in S.1 Grid

1a Pleasant
1b Vicious, hard
2a Friendly
2b Antagonistic
3a Intelligent, have depth of character
3b Superficial
4a Serious
4b Relaxed
5a Like me
5b Not like me
6a Like to be liked
6b Not concerned about whether people like them or not
7a Interesting
7b Not interesting
8a Worry about things unnecessarily

8b Do not worry about things unnecessarily
9a Do not have peace of mind
9b Have peace of mind
10a Tolerant
10b Intolerant
11a Listen to others' point of view
11b Do not listen to others' point of view
12a Have good relations with others
12b Do not have good relations with others
13a Stutterers
13b Normal speakers
14a Like I'd like to be
14b Not like I'd like to be
15a Have feelings of inferiority
15b Do not have feelings of inferiority
16a Respected
16b Not respected

Constructs in S.2 Grid

1a Lack confidence
1b Confident
2a Earnest
2b Relaxed
3a Ordinary
3b Distinguished
4a Intelligent
4b Unintelligent
5a Depth of character
5b Vacant
6a Like me in character
6b Not like me in character
7a Do not live life to the full
7b Have opportunity to live life to the full
8a Envious
8b Not envious
9a Sober, conscious of his particular status symbol
9b Not concerned with impressing people
10a Do not relax and laugh much
10b Happy with status in life
11a May or may not be respected
11b Always respected
12a Feel inferior
12b Feel superior
13a Have understanding of a lot of things
13b Do not have understanding of a lot of things
14a Deeper enjoyment of life
14b No depth of enjoyment of life
15a Stutterers
15b Fluent speaker

CONSTRUCTS IN S.3 GRID

1a Lack confidence
1b Confident
2a Desire to please, not to offend
2b Do not consider it important to please all the time
3a Serious
3b Gay, light-hearted
4a Like me in character
4b Not like me in character
5a Pitied
5b Liked
6a Make no definite impression
6b Make a definite impression
7a Do not necessarily get on well with people
7b Get on well with people
8a Have increased chance of being liked
8b Do not consider it important to be liked
9a Cannot handle situations in which is disliked
9b Can handle situation in which is disliked
10a Not interested in making friends
10b Interested in making friends
11a Stutterers
11b Fluent person
12a Less easy to get to know
12b Easy to get to know

CONSTRUCTS IN S.4 GRID

1a Self confident
1b Lack self confidence
2a Socially odd
2b Socially acceptable
3a Lack of sense of humour
3b Have a sense of humour
4a Like me in character
4b Not like me in character
5a Have a feeling of well-being
5b Do not have a feeling of well-being
6a Not seen as their true self
6b Seen as their true self, for what they are
7a Less liked by people
7b Liked more by people
8a Do not believe that society would break down if people were angry with each other
8b Believe that society would break down if people were angry with each other
9a Stutterers
9b Mentally and physically fluent person

References

Adams, M. R. (1969). "Psychological Differences Between Stutterers and Non-stutterers: a Review of the Experimental Literature." *J. Comm. Dis.*, **2**, 163–170.

Albright, M. A. H. and Malone, J. Y. (1942). "The Relationship of Hearing Acuity to Stammering." *J. Except. Children*, **8**, 186–190.

Allport, G. W. (1940). "Liberalism and the Motives of Men." *In* "Frontiers of Democracy." Vol. 6. pp. 136–137.

Allport, G. W. (1964). "The Fruits of Eclecticism—Bitter or Sweet?" *Acta Psychol.*, **23**, 27–44.

Anastasi, A. (1958). "Differential Psychology." (3rd ed.) Macmillan, New York.

Andrews, G. and Harris, M. (1964). "The Syndrome of Stuttering." Spastic Soc. Med. Educ. Inf., Heinemann, London.

Appelt, A. (1911). "The Real Cause of Stammering and Its Permanent Cure." Methuen, London

Aron, Myrtle (1962). "The Nature and Incidence of Stuttering Among a Bantu Group of School-Going Children." *J. Speech Hear. Disorders*, **27**, 116–128.

Bachrach, D. L. (1964). "Sex Differences in Reactions to Delayed Auditory Feedback." *Percept. Mot. Skills*, **19**, 81–82.

Bacon, F. (1627). "Sylva Sylvarum or Natural History in Ten Centuries." Century IV, Sect. 386.

Baloff, N. and Becker, S. W. (1967). "On the Futility of Aggregating Individual Learning Curves." *Psychol. Rep.*, **20**, 183–191.

Bannister, D. (1959). "An Application of Personal Construct Theory (Kelly) to Schizoid Thinking." Unpublished Ph.D. thesis, University of London.

Bannister, D. (1960). "Conceptual Structure in Thought Disordered Schizophrenics." *J. ment. Sci.*, **106**, 1230–1249.

Bannister, D. (1962). "The Nature and Measurement of Schizophrenic Thought Disorder." *J. ment. Sci.*, **108**, 825–842.

Bannister, D. (1963). "The Genesis of Schizophrenic Thought Disorder: a Serial Invalidation Hypothesis." *Br. J. Psychiat.*, **109**, 680–686.

Bannister, D. and Fransella, Fay, (1966). "A Grid Test of Schizophrenic Thought Disorder." *Br. J. Soc. clin. Psychol.*, **5**, 95–102.

Bannister, D. and Fransella, Fay, (1967). "A Grid Test of Schizophrenic Thought Disorder." Psychological Test Publications, Barnstaple.

Bannister, D. and Fransella, Fay, (1971). "Inquiring Man: the Theory of Personal Constructs." Penguin Books, London.

Bannister, D. and Mair, J. M. M. (1968). "The Evaluation of Personal Constructs." Academic Press, London and New York.

Bannister, D. and Salmon, Phillida, (1967). "Measures of Superordinacy." Unpublished study.

Barbara, D. A. (1958). "Stuttering: a Psychodynamic Approach to its Understanding and Treatment." Hutchinson, London.

Beech, H. R. (1969). "Changing Man's Behaviour." Penguin Books, London.

Beech, H. R. and Fransella, Fay, (1968). "Research and Experiment in Stuttering." Pergamon Press, London.

Beech, H. R. and Fransella, Fay, (1969). "Explanations of the 'Rhythm Effect' in Stuttering." *In* "Stuttering and the Conditioning Therapies" (B. B. Gray and G. England, eds.), Monterey Speech and Hearing Institute, California.

Bender, J. (1942). "The Stuttering Personality." *Am. J. Orthopsychiat.*, **12**, 140–146.

Berlin, C. I. (1960). "Parents' Diagnoses of Stuttering." *J. Speech Hear. Disorders*, **3**, 372–379.

Biggs, Barbara and Sheehan, J. G. (1969). "Punishment or Distraction? Operant Stuttering Revisited." *J. abnorm. Psychol.*, **74**, 256–262.

Blackburn, W. B. (1931). "Study of Voluntary Movements in Stutterers and Normal Speakers." *Psychol. Monogr.*, **41**, 1–13.

Bloodstein, O. (1949). "Conditions under which Stuttering is Reduced or Absent: a Review of the Literature." *J. Speech Hear. Disorders*, **14**, 295–302.

Bloodstein, O. (1969). "A Handbook on Stuttering." National Easter Seal Society for Crippled Children and Adults, Chicago.

Bloodstein, O. and Schreiber, L. R. (1957). "Obsessive-Compulsive Reactions in Stutterers." *J. Speech Hear. Disorders*, **22**, 33–39.

Bluemel, C. S. (1957). "The Riddle of Stuttering". Instate Publishing Co., Danville, U.S.A.

Bonarius, J. C. J. (1965). "Research in the Personal Construct Theory of George A. Kelly: Role Construct Repertory Test and Basic Theory." *In* "Progress in Experimental Personality Research", (B. Maher, ed.), Academic Press, New York and London.

Bourdon, Karen H. and Silber, D. E. (1970). "Perceived Parental Behaviour among Stutterers and Nonstutterers." *J. abnorm. Psychol.*, **75**, 93–97.

Brady, J. P. (1968). "A Behavioural Approach to the Treatment of Stuttering." *Am. J. Psychiat.*, **125**, 843–848.

Brady, J. P. (1969). "Studies on the Metronome Effect on Stuttering." *Behav. Res. Ther.*, **7**, 197–204.

Brady, J. P. (1971). "Metronome-Conditioned Speech Retraining for Stuttering." *Behav. Ther.*, **2**, 129–150.

Brandon, S. and Harris, Mary, (1967). "Stammering—an Experimental Treatment Programme using Syllable-Timed-Speech." *Br. J. Dis. Comm.*, **2**, 64–68.

Broen, Patricia and Siegel, G. M. (1972). "Variations in Normal Speech Disfluencies." *Language and Speech*. (In press).

Brown, S. F. (1945). "The Loci of Stutterings in the Speech Sequence." *J. Speech Hear. Disorders*, **10**, 181–192.

Brutten, E. J. (1963). "Palmar Sweat Investigation of Disfluency and Expectancy Adaptation." *J. Speech Hear. Disorders*, **6**, 40–48.

Brutten, E. J. and Shoemaker, D. J. (1967). "The Modification of Stuttering." Englewood Cliffs, Prentice-Hall, New Jersey.

Cherry, C. and Sayers, B. McA. (1956). "Experiments Upon the Total Inhibition of Stammering by External Control, and Some Clinical Results". *J. psychosom. Res.*, **1**, 233–246.

Colombat de l'Isere. (1840). "Du Begaiement et de tous les autres Vices de la Parole Traites par de Nouvelles Methodes." (3rd ed.) Manut Fils, Paris.

Conant, J. B. (1951). "Science and Common Sense," Yale University Press, New Haven.

Conlon, Sara. (1966). "Attitudes of Adults Toward Themselves and Those Who Stutter." *Diss. Abstr.*, **27**, 841–842.

Cooper, Crystal and Cooper, E. B. (1969). "Variations in Adult Stutterer Attitudes Towards Clinicians During Therapy." *J. Comm. Dis.*, **2**, 141–153.

Cooper, E. B. (1965). "An Inquiry into the Use of Inter-Personal Communications as a Source of Therapy for Stutterers." *In* "New Directions in Stuttering," (D. Barbara, ed.) Charles C. Thomas, Springfield, Illinois, U.S.A.

Cross, H. M. (1936). "The Motor Capacities of Stutterers." *Archives of Speech*, **1**, 112–132.

Curlee, R. F. and Perkins, W. H. (1969). "The Effects of Punishment of Expectancies to Stutter on the Frequencies of Subsequent Expectancies and Stuttering." *J. Speech Hear. Disorders*, **11**, 787–795.

Darwin, Erasmus, (1801). "Zoonomia: or the Laws of Organic Life." J. Johnson, London. (3rd ed.).

Delia, J. G., Gonyea, A. H. and Crockett, W. H. (1971). "The Effects of Subject-Generated and Normative Constructs Upon the Formation of Impressions." *Br. J. soc. clin. Psychol.*, **10**, 301–305.

Dieffenbach, J. F. (1841). "Memoir on the Radical Cure of Stuttering by Surgical Operation." Translated by Joseph Travers, London.

Dixon, C. (1947). "The Amount and Rate of Adaptation of Stuttering in Different Oral Reading Situations." M.A. thesis, State University of Iowa.

Douglass, E. and Quarrington, B. (1952). "The Differentiation of Interiorized and Exteriorized Secondary Stuttering." *J. Speech Hear. Disorders*, **17**, 377–385.

Eisenson, J. (1966). "Observations of the Incidence of Stuttering in a Special Culture." *J. Am. Speech Hear. Assoc.*, **8**, 391–394.

Eldridge, Margaret, (1968). "The History of the Treatment of Speech Disorders." E. S. Livingstone Ltd., Edinburgh and London.

Ellis, A. (1962). "Reason and Emotion in Psychotherapy." Lyle Stuart, New York.

English, H. B. and English, Ava, (1958). "A Comprehensive Dictionary of Psychological and Psychoanalytical Terms." Longmans, New York.

Epting, F. R., Suchman, D. I. and Nickeson, C. J. (1971). "An Evaluation of Elicitation Procedures for Personal Constructs." *Br. J. Psychol.*, **62**, 513–517.

Fiedler, F. E. and Wepman, J. (1951). "An Exploratory Investigation of the Self Concept of Stutterers." *J. Speech Hear. Disorders*, **16**, 110–114.

Finkelstein, P. and Weisberger, S. (1954). "The Motor Proficiency of Stutterers." *J. Speech Hear. Disorders*, **19**, 52–58.

Flanagan, B., Goldiamond, I. and Azrin, N. H. (1958). "Operant Stuttering: the Control of Stuttering Through Response-Contingent Consequences." *J. Exp. analysis Behav.*, **1**, 173–177.

Forster, E. S. (1927). "The Works of Aristotle." Clarendon Press, Oxford.

Fransella, Fay, (1965a). "The Effects of Imposed Rhythm and Certain Aspects of Personality on the Speech of Stutterers." Unpublished Ph.D. thesis, University of London.

Fransella, Fay, (1965b). "An Experimental Evaluation of the Speech Correction Semantic Differential." *Speech Monogr.*, **32**, 448–451.

Fransella, Fay, (1967). "Rhythm as a Distractor in the Modification of Stuttering." *Behav. Res. Ther.*, **5**, 253–255.

Fransella, Fay, (1968). "Self Concepts and the Stutterer." *Br. J. Psychiat.*, **114**, 1531–1535.

Fransella, Fay, (1969). "The Stutterer as Subject or Object?" *In* "Stuttering and the Conditioning Therapies." (B. B. Gray and G. England, eds.), Monterey Institute for Speech and Hearing, California.

Fransella, Fay, (1970a). "Stuttering: Not a Symptom but a Way of Life." *Br. J. comm. Dis.*, **5**, 22–29.

Fransella, Fay, (1970b). ". . . And Then There Was One." *In* "Perspectives in Personal Construct Theory." (D. Bannister, ed.), Academic Press, London and New York.

Fransella, Fay, (1970c). "Measurement of Conceptual Change Accompanying Weight Loss." *Psychosom. Res.* **14**, 347–351.

Fransella, Fay. (1971a). "The 'Rhythm Effect' in Stuttering as a Function of Predictability of Utterance." *Behav. Res. Ther.*, **9**, 265–271.

Fransella, Fay, (1971b). "A Personal Construct Theory and Treatment of Stuttering." *J. Psychosom. Res.*, **15**, 433–438.

Fransella, Fay, (1972). "Thinking in the Obsessional." *In* "Obsessional Disorder." (H. R. Beech, ed.), Methuen, London (in press).

Fransella, Fay and Adams, B. (1966). "An Illustration of the Use of Repertory Grid Technique in a Clinical Setting." *Br. J. soc. clin. Psychol.*, **5**, 51–62.

Fransella, Fay and Bannister, D. (1967). "A Validation of Repertory Grid Technique as a Measure of Political Construing." *Acta Psychol.*, **26**, 97–106.

Fransella, Fay and Beech, H. R. (1965). "An Experimental Analysis of the Effect of Rhythm on the Speech of Stutterers." *Behav. Res. Ther.*, **3**, 195–201.

Fransella, Fay and Crisp, A. H. (1970). "Conceptual Organization and Weight Change." *Psychosom. Psychother*, **18**, 176–185. Reprinted in "Recent Research in Psychosomatics." (R. A. Pierloot, ed.), S. Karger, Basel, 1971.

Fransella, Fay and Joyston-Bechal, M. P. (1971). "An Investigation of Conceptual Process and Pattern Change in a Psychotherapy Group." *Br. J. Psychiat.*, **119**, 199–206.

French, P. (1966). "The Stammerer as Hero," *Encounter*, **27**, 67–75.

Goldiamond, I. (1965). "Stuttering and Fluency as Manipulative Operant Response Classes." *In* "Research in Behaviour Modification." (L. Krasner and L. P. Ullman, eds.), Holt, Rinehart and Winston, New York.

Goldiamond, I. (1969). "Psychological Problems as Disrupting Operants Rather than Disrupted Behaviours: Implications for Analysis and Treatment." *Proc. Internat. Congr. Psychol.*, London.

Goldman, R. (1965). "The Effects of Cultural Patterns on the Sex Ratio in Stuttering." *J. Am. Speech Hear. Assoc.*, abstract, **7**, 370.

Goldman, R. and Shames, G. H. (1964a). "A Study of Goal-Setting Behaviour of Parents of Stutterers and Parents of Nonstutterers." *J. Speech Hear. Res.*, **29**, 192–194.

Goldman, R. and Shames, G. H. (1964b). "Comparisons of the Goals that Parents of Stutterers and Parents of Nonstutterers Set For Their Children." *J. Speech Hear. Disorders*, **29**, 381–389.

Goldman-Eisler, F. (1958). "Speech Production and the Probability of Words in Context." *Q. J. Exp. Psychol.*, **10**, 96–106.

Goodstein, L. D. (1958). "Functional Speech Disorders and Personality: a Survey of the Research." *J. Speech Hear. Disorders*, **1**, 359–376.

Gray, B. B. (1965). "Theoretical Approximations of Stuttering Adaptation." *Behav. Res. Ther.*, **3**, 171–185.

Gray, B. B. and Karmen, Jane, (1967). "The Relationship Between Nonverbal Anxiety and Stuttering Adaptation." *J. Comm. Dis.*, **1**, 141–151.

Gregory, H. H. (1964). "Stuttering and Auditory Central Nervous System Disorder." *J. Speech Hear. Disorders*, **7**, 335–341.

Gregory, H. H. (1969). "An Assessment of the Results of Stuttering Therapy." Final Report, Research and Demonstration Project 1725-S, Social and Rehabilitation Service, U.S. Dept. of H.E. and W.

Hackett, J. D., Hoffman, M., MacLeod, A. W. and Surtees, R. (1958). "A Study of the Effects of Chlorpromazine as an Aid to Therapy for Stuttering with a One-Year Follow-Up." *J. Am. Speech Hear. Assoc.*, abstract.

Halle, (1900). "Ueber Störungen der Athmung bei Stottern." *Monatshr. Sprachheilkunde*, **10**, 225.

Hejna, R. (1960). "Speech Disorders and Non-Directive Therapy." Ronald Press, New York.

Hill, H. (1944). "Stuttering: 1. A Critical Review and Evaluation of Biochemical Investigations." *J. Speech Hear Disorders*, **9**, 245–261.

Hinkle, D. E. (1965). "The Change of Personal Constructs From the Viewpoint of a Theory of Implications." Unpublished Ph.D. thesis, Ohio State University.

Holz, W. C. and Azrin, N. H. (1961). "Discriminative Properties of Punishment." *J. exp. analysis Behav.*, **4**, 225–232.

Hoy, R. M. (1972) "The Meaning of Alcoholism for Alcoholics." *Br. J. soc. clin. Psychol.*, (in press).

Hunsley, Y. L. (1937). "Dysintegration in the Speech Musculature of Stutterers During the Production of a Nonverbal Temporal Pattern." *Psychol. Monogr.*, **49**, 32–49.

Ingham, R. J. and Andrews, G. (1972a). "The Relation Between Anxiety Reduction and Treatment." Unpublished manuscript.

Ingham, R. J. and Andrews, G. (1972b). "Stuttering: A Comparison of the Effectiveness of Four Treatment Techniques." *J. Comm, Dis.*, **5**, 91–117.

Ingham, R. J. and Andrews, G. (1972c). "The Quality of Fluency After Treatment." Unpublished manuscript.

Jasper, H. H. (1932). "A Laboratory Study of Diagnostic Indices of Bilateral Neuromuscular Organization in Stutterers and Normal Speakers." *Psychol. Monogr.*, **43**, 72–174.

Johnson, D. T. and Spielberger, C. D. (1968). "The Effects of Relaxation Training and the Passage of Time on Measures of State and Trait Anxiety." *J. clin. Psychol.*, **24**, 20–23.

Johnson, W. (1955). "A Study of the Onset and Development of Stuttering." *In* "Stuttering in Children and Adults." (Johnson, W. and Leutenegger, R. R., eds.), University of Minnesota Press, Minneapolis.

Johnson, W. and Knott, J. (1937). "Studies in the Psychology of Stuttering; 1. The Distribution of Moments of Stuttering in Successive Readings of the Same Material." *J. Speech Hear Disorders*, **2**, 17–19.

Johnson, W., Stearns, G. and Warweg, E. (1933). "Chemical Factors and the Stuttering Spasm." *Q. J. Speech*, **19**, 409–414.

Johnson, W., Brown, S. F., Curtis, J. F., Edney, C. W. and Keaster, J. (1956). "Speech Handicapped School Children." Harper and Row, New York. 2nd edition.

Johnson, W., Young, M. A., Sahs, A. L. and Dedell, G. N. (1959). "Effects of Hyperventilation and Tetany on the Speech Fluency of Stutterers and Nonstutterers." *J. Speech Hear. Disorders*, **2**, 203–215.

Johnson, W., Darley, F. L. and Spriestersbach, D. C. (1963). "Diagnostic Methods in Speech Pathology." Harper and Row, New York.

Johnson, W., Brown, S. F., Curtis, J. F., Edney, C. W. and Keaster, J. (1967). "Speech Handicapped School Children." Harper and Row, New York. 3rd edition.

Jones, R. K. (1966). "Observations on Stammering After Localized Cerebral Injury." *J. Neurol. Neurosurg. Psychiat.*, **29**, 192–195.

Karlin, I. W. and Sorbel, A. E. (1940). "A Comprehensive Study of the Blood Chemistry of Stutterers and Nonstutterers." *Speech Monogr.*, **7**, 75–84.

Kastein, S. (1947). "The Chewing Method of Treating Stuttering." *J. Speech Hear. Disorders*, **12**, 195–198.

Kelly, G. A. (1932). "Some Common Factors in Reading and Speech Disabilities." *Psychol. Monogr.*, **43**, 175–203.

Kelly, G. A. (1955). "The Psychology of Personal Constructs." Norton, New York.

Kelly, G. A. (1962). "Europe's Matrix of Decision." *In* "Nebraska Symposium on Motivation." (M. R. Jones, ed.), University of Nebraska Press, Lincoln.

Kelly, G. A. (1970). "Behaviour is an Experiment." *In* "Perspectives in Personal Construct Theory." (D. Bannister, ed.), Academic Press, London and New York.

Kendall, M. G. and Stuart, A. (1969). "The Advanced Theory of Statistics." Griffin, London.

Kent, Louise, (1963). "The Use of Tranquilizers in the Treatment of Stuttering." *J. Speech Hear. Disorders*, **28**, 288–294.

Kern, A. (1932). "Der Einfluss des Hörens auf des Stottern." *Arch. Psychiat. Nervkrankh.*, **97**, 429–449.

Klencke, H. (1844). "Die Stoerungen des Menschlicken Stimm-und-Sprachorgans." Kassel.

Knowles, J. B. and Purves, S. C. (1965). "The Use of Repertory Grid Technique to Assess the Influence of the Experimenter-Subject Relationship in Verbal Conditioning." *Bull. Br. psychol. Soc.*, **18**, 59.

Kŏndas, O. (1969). "Shadowing Technique in the Treatment of Stammering and Reading Disability." *Proc. Internat. Congr. Psychol.*, London.

Kopp, G. A. (1934). "Metabolic Studies of Stutterers. I. Biochemical Study of Blood Composition." *Speech Monogr.*, **1**, 117–130.

Kopp, Helene, (1943). "The Relationship of Stuttering to Motor Disturbances." *Nerv. Child*, **2**, 107–116.

Krugman, M. (1946). "Psychosomatic Study of Fifty Stuttering Children. Round Table IV, Rorschach Study." *Am. J. Orthopsychiat.*, **16**, 127–133.

Laing, R. D. (1967). "The Politics of Experience." Penguin Books, London.

Landfield, A. W. (1954). "A Movement Interpretation of Threat." *J. abnorm. soc. Psychol.*, **40**, 529–532.

Landfield, A. W. (1965). "Role Construct Scoring Manual." Unpublished manuscript.

Landfield, A. W. (1967). "Revised Role Construct Scoring Manual." Unpublished manuscript.

Landfield, A. W. (1971). "Personal Construct Systems in Psychotherapy." McNally Rand, New York.

Landfield, A. W. and Fjeld, P. (1960). "Threat and Self Predictability with Predictability of Others Controlled: an Addendum." *Psychol. Rep.*, **6**, 333–334.

Langova, J. and Moravek, M. (1964). "Some Results of Experimental Examinations Among Stutterers and Clutterers." *Folia Phoniat.*, **16**, 290–296.

Lanyon, R. L. (1965). "The relationship of Adaptation and Consistency to Improvement in Stuttering Therapy." *J. Speech Hear. Disorders*, **8**, 263–269.

Lanyon, R. L. (1969). "Behaviour Change in Stuttering Through Systematic Desensitization." *J. Speech Hear. Disorders*, **34**, 253–260.

Lee, B. S. (1951). "Artificial Stutter." *J. Speech Hear. Disorders*, **16**, 53–55.

Lemert, E. M. (1962). "Stuttering and Social Structure in Two Pacific Societies." *J. Speech Hear. Disorders*, **27**, 3–10.

Levy, L. H. (1956). "Personal Constructs and Predictive Behaviour." *J. abnorm. soc. Psychol.*, **53**, 54–58.

Love, W. R. (1955). "The Effect of Pentobarbital (Nembutal) and Amphetamine Sulphate (Benzedrine) on the Severity of Stuttering." *In* "Stuttering in Children and Adults." (W. Johnson, ed.) Minnesota Press, Minneapolis.

Madison, L. R. and Norman, R. D. (1952). "A Comparison of the Performance of Stutterers and Nonstutterers on the Rosenzweig Picture-Frustration Test." *J. clin. Psychol.*, **8**, 179–183.

Mair, J. M. M. (1964). "The Derivation, Reliability and Validity of Grid Measures. Some Problems and Suggestions." *Bull. Br. psychol. Soc.*, **17**, 55.

Mair, J. M. M. (1966). "Prediction of Grid Scores." *Br. J. Psychol.*, **57**, 187–192.

Manning, W. H. and Cooper, E. B. (1969). "Variations in Attitudes of the Adult Stutterer Toward His Clinician Related to Progress in Therapy." *J. Comm. Dis.*, **2**, 154–162.

Maraist, J. A. and Hutton, C. (1957). "Effects of Auditory Masking Upon the Speech of Stutterers." *J. Speech Hear. Disorders*, **22**, 385–389.

Martin, R. R. and Haroldson, S. K. (1969). "The Effects of Two Treatment Procedures on Stuttering." *J. Comm. Dis.*, **2**, 115–125.

Martyn, Margaret, Sheehan, J. G. and Schultz, Karen, (1969). "Incidence of Stuttering and Other Speech Disorders Among the Retarded." *Amer. J. Ment. Def.*, **74**, 206–211.

McCrosky, R. (1957). "Effect of Speech on Metabolism: a Comparison Between Stutterers and Nonstutterers." *J. Speech Hear. Disorders* **22**, 46–52.

McDearmon, J. R. (1968). "Primary Stuttering at the Onset of Stuttering: A Reexamination of the Data." *J. Speech Hear. Disorders*, **11**, 631–637.

Meyer, V. and Comley, J. (1967). "A Preliminary Report on the Treatment of Stammer by the Use of Rhythmic Stimulation." *In* "Stuttering and the Conditioning Therapies." (B. B. Gray and G. England, eds.), Monterey Speech and Hearing Institute, California.

Meyer, V. and Mair, J. M. M. (1963). "A New Technique to Control Stammering: a Preliminary Report." *Behav. Res. Ther.*, **1**, 251–254.

Milisen, R. (1957). "Methods of Evaluation and Diagnosis of Speech Disorders." *In* "Handbook of Speech Pathology." (L. E. Travis, ed.), Appleton-Century-Crofts Inc., New York.

Mitchell, B. A. (1955). "An Analysis of the Effect of Reserpine on Adult Stutterers." Unpublished M.A. dissertation, Western Michigan University.

Moravek, M. and Langova, A. (1962). "Some Electrophysiological Findings Among Stutterers and Clutterers." *Folia phoniat.*, **14**, 395–416.

Morley, D. E. (1957). "The Development and Disorders of Speech in Childhood." Livingstone, Edinburgh.

Morgenstern, J. (1956). "Socio-Economic Factors in Stuttering." *J. Speech Hear. Disorders*, **21**, 25–33.

Neelley, J. (1961). "A Study of the Speech of Stutterers and Nonstutterers

Under Normal and Delayed Auditory Feedback." *J. Speech Hear. Disorders, Monogr. Suppl.*, **7**, 63–82.

Neelley, J. and Timmons, R. (1967). "Adaptation and Consistency in the Disfluent Speech Behaviour of Young Stutterers and Nonstutterers." *J. Speech Hear. Res.*, **10**, 250–256.

Orton, S. T. (1927). "Studies in Stuttering." *Arch. Neurol. Psychiat. Lond.*, **18**, 671–672.

Owen, T. and Stemmermann, P. (1947). "Electric Convulsive Therapy in Stammering." *J. Psychiat.*, **104**, 410–413.

Payne, D. E. (1956). "Role Constructs *Versus* Part Constructs and Interpersonal Understanding." Unpublished Ph.D. dissertation, Ohio State University.

Prins, D. (1968). "Pre-Therapy Adaptation of Stuttering and Its Relation to Speech Measures of Therapy Progress." *J. Speech Hear. Disorders*, **11**, 740–746.

Quarrington, B. (1965). "Stuttering as a Function of the Information Value and Sentence Position of Words." *J. abnorm. Psychol.*, **70**, 221–224.

Quarrington, B. and Douglass, E. (1960). "Audibility Avoidance in Nonvocalized Stutterers." *J. Speech Hear. Disorders*, **25**, 358–365.

Quarrington, B., Conway, J. K. and Siegel, N. (1962). "An Experimental Study of Some Properties of Stuttered Words." *J. Speech Hear. Res.*, **5**, 388–394.

Quarrington, B., Seligman, Judy and Kosower, Eleanor, (1969). "Goal Setting Behaviour of Parents of Beginning Stutterers and Parents of Nonstuttering Children." *J. Speech Hear. Disorders*, **12**, 435–442.

Rieber, R. W. and Froeschels, E. (1966). "An Historical Review of the European Literature in Speech Pathology." *In* "Speech Pathology." (R. W. Rieber and R. S. Brubaker, eds.), North-Holland Publishing Co., Amsterdam.

Rogers, C. (1961). "On Becoming a Person." Houghton Mifflin, Boston.

Rotter, J. B. (1955). "A Study of the Motor Integration of Stutterers and Nonstutterers." *In* "Stuttering in Children and Adults." (W. Johnson, ed.), University of Minnesota Press, Minneapolis.

Salmon, Phillida, (1963). "A Clinical Investigation of Sexual Identity." Unpublished case study.

Salmon, Phillida, (1970). "A Psychology of Personal Growth." *In* "Perspectives in Personal Construct Theory." (D. Bannister, ed.), Academic Press, London and New York.

Sander, E. K. (1961). "Reliability of the Iowa Speech Disfluency Test." *J. Speech Hear. Disorders, Monogr. Suppl.*, **7**, 21–30.

Sander, E. K. (1963). "Frequency of Syllable Repetitions and 'Stutterer' Judgements." *J. Speech Hear. Disorders*, **28**, 19–30.

Sander, E. K. (1965). "Comments on Investigating Listener Reactions to Speech Disfluency." *J. Speech Hear. Disorders*, **30**, 159–165.

Santostefano, S. (1960). "Anxiety and Hostility." *J. Speech Hear Res.*, **3**, 337–347.

Sayles, D. G. (1967). "Brain-Wave Excitability, Perseveration and Stuttering." *Diss. Abstr.*, **27**, (19-B) 3328.

Schlanger, B. B. and Gottsleben, R. H. (1957). "Analysis of Speech Defects Among the Institutionalized Mentally Retarded." *J. Speech Hear. Disorders*, **22**, 98–103.

Schuell, H. (1946). "Sex Differences in Relation to Stuttering." *J. Speech Hear. Disorders*, **11**, 277–298.

Seeman, M. (1966). "Speech Pathology in Czechoslovakia." *In* "Speech Pathology." (R. W. Rieber and R. S. Brubaker, eds.), North-Holland Publishing Co., Amsterdam.

Shames, G. H., Egolf, D. B. and Rhodes, R. C. (1969). "Experimental Programs in Stuttering Therapy." *J. Speech Hear. Disorders*, **34**, 30–47.

Shane, M. L. (1955). "Effect on Stuttering of Alteration in Auditory Feedback." *In* "Stuttering in Children and Adults." (W. Johnson, ed.), University of Minnesota Press, Minneapolis.

Shapiro, M. B. (1961). "The Single Case in Fundamental Clinical Psychological Research." *Br. J. Med. Psychol.*, **34**, 255–262.

Shapiro, M. B. (1964). "The Measurement of Clinically Relevant Variables." *J. Psychosom. Res.*, **8**, 245–254.

Shearer, W. M. (1961). "A Theoretical Consideration of the Self-Concept and Body-Image in Stuttering Therapy." *J. Am. Speech Hear. Assoc.*, **3**, 115–116.

Shearer, W. M. and Simmons, F. B. (1965). "Middle Ear Activity During Speech in Normal Speakers and Stutterers." *J. Speech Hear. Res.*, **8**, 203–207.

Sheehan, J. G. (1954). "An Integration of Psychotherapy and Speech Therapy Through a Conflict Theory of Stuttering." *J. Speech Hear. Disorders*, **19**, 474–482.

Sheehan, J. G. (1958). "Projective Studies of Stuttering." *J. Speech Hear. Disorders*, **23**, 18–25.

Sheehan, J. G. (1969). "Cyclic Variation in Stuttering: Comment on Taylor and Taylor's 'Test of Predictions From the Conflict Hypothesis of Stuttering'." *J. abnorm. Psychol.*, **74**, 452–453.

Sheehan, J. G. (1970). "Stuttering: Research and Therapy." Harper and Row, New York.

Sheehan, J. G. and Martyn, Margaret, (1966). "Spontaneous Recovery From Stuttering." *J. Speech Hear. Res.*, **9**, 121–135.

Sheehan, J. G. and Martyn, Margaret, (1970). "Stuttering and Its Disappearance." *J. Speech Hear. Res.*, **13**, 279–289.

Sheehan, J. G. and Zelen, S. L. (1955). "Level of Aspiration in Stutterers and Non-stutterers." *J. abnorm. soc. Psychol.*, **51**, 83–86.

Sheehan, J. G., Martyn, Margaret, and Kilburn, K. K. (1968). "Speech Disorders in Retardation." *Am. J. ment. Def.*, **73**, 251–256.

Sheridan, T. (1762). "A Course of Lectures on Elocution." W. Strahan and A. Millar, London.

Siegel, G. M. and Martin, R. R. (1965a). "Experimental Modification of Disfluency in Normal Speakers." *J. Speech Hear. Res.*, **8**, 236–244.

Siegel, G. M. and Martin, R. R. (1965b). "Verbal Punishment of Disfluencies in Normal Speakers." *J. Speech Hear. Res.*, **8**, 245–251.

Silverman, F. H. and Williams, D. E. (1967). "Loci of Disfluencies in the Speech of Nonstutterers During Oral Reading." *J. Speech Hear. Res.*, **10**, 790–794.

Slater, P. (1965). "The Principal Components of a Repertory Grid." Vincent Andrews and Co., London.

Smith, R. G. (1962). "A Semantic Differential for Speech Correction Concepts." *Speech Monogr.*, **29**, 32–37.

Spriestersbach, D. C. (1940). "An Exploratory Study of the Motility of the Peripheral Oral Structures in Relation to Defective and Superior Consonant Articulation." M.A. thesis, State University of Iowa.

Ssikorski, J. A. (1894). "About Stammering." (original in Russian).

Starr, H. E. (1922). "The Hydrogen Ion Concentration of the Mixed Saliva, Considered as an Index of Fatigue and of Emotional Excitement and Applied to the Study of the Metabolic Etiology of Stammering." *Am. J. Psychol.*, **33**, 394–418.

Starr, H. E. (1928). "Psychological Concomitants of Higher Alveolar Carbon Dioxide: a Psychobiochemical Study of the Etiology of Stammering." *Psychol. Clinic*, **17**, 1–12.

Stewart, J. L. (1960). "The Problem of Stuttering in Certain North American Indian Societies." *J. Speech Hear. Disorders, Monogr. Suppl.*, **6**, 1–87.

Sutton, S. and Chase, R. A. (1961). "White Noise and Stuttering." *J. Speech Hear. Res.*, **4**, 72.

Taylor, I. (1966a). "The Properties of Stuttered Words." *J. Verb. Learn. Verb. Behav.*, **5**, 112–118.

Taylor, I. (1966b). "What Words Are Stuttered?" *Psychol. Bull.*, **65**, 233–242.

Thelwell, J. (1810). "A Letter to Henry Cline, Esquire, on Imperfect Development of the Faculties, Mental and Moral, as Well as Constitutional and Organic; and on the Treatment of Impediments of Speech." London.

Thomé. (1867). "Pathologie und Therapie des Stotterns."

Travis, L. E. (1927). "Dysintegration of Breathing Movements During Stuttering." *Arch. Neurol. Psychiat.*, **18**, 672–690.

Travis, L. E. (1931). "Speech Pathology." Appleton-Century, New York.

Trotter, W. D. and Kools, J. A. (1955). "Listener Adaptation to the Severity of Stuttering." *J. Speech Hear. Disorders*, **20**, 385–387.

Van Dantzig, B. (1939). "Writing, Typing and Speaking." *J. Speech Hear. Disorders*, **4**, 297–301.

Van Dantzig, M. (1940). "Syllable-Tapping, a New Method For the Help of Stammerers." *J. Speech Hear. Disorders*, **5**, 127–131.

Van Riper, C. (1936). "Study of the Thoracic Breathing of Stutterers During Expectancy and Occurrence of Stuttering Spasms." *J. Speech Hear. Disorders*, **I**, 61–72.

Van Riper, C. (1954). "Speech Correction: Principles and Methods." (3rd edition) Prentice-Hall, New Jersey.

Van Riper, C. (1958). "Experiments in Stuttering Therapy." *In* "Stuttering: A Symposium." (J. Eisenson, ed.), Harper and Row, New York.

Van Riper, C. (1971). "The Nature of Stuttering." Prentice-Hall, New Jersey.

Wallen, V. (1959). "A Q-Technique Study of Self-Concepts of Adolescent Stutterers and Nonstutterers." Ph.D. dissertation, Boston University.

Walnut, A. (1954). "A Personality Inventory Item Analysis of Individuals Who Stutter and Individuals Who Have Other Handicaps." *J. Speech Hear. Disorders*, **19**, 220–227.

Walter, W. G. (1961). "The Living Brain." Penguin Books, London.

Webster, R. L. (1970). "Stuttering: A Way to Eliminate It and a Way to Explain It." *In* "Control of Human Behaviour." Vol. 2. (R. Ulrich, T. Stachnik and J. Mabry, eds.), Scott, Foresman and Co., Illinois.

Wells, P. G. and Malcolm, M. T. (1971). "Controlled Trial of the Treatment of 36 Stutterers." *Br. J. Psychiat.*, **119**, 603–604.

Wendhal, R. W. and Cole, J. (1961). "Identification of Stuttering During Relatively Fluent Speech." *J. Speech Hear. Disorders*, **4**, 281–286.

Williams, D. E. and Kent, Louise, (1958). "Listener Evaluations of Speech Interruptions." *J. Speech Hear. Res.*, **I**, 124–131.

Williams, D. E., Silverman, F. H. and Kools, J. A. (1968). "Disfluency Behaviour of Elementary School Stutterers and Nonstutterers: the Adaptation Effect." *J. Speech Hear. Res.*, **11**, 622–730.

Williams, D. E., Silverman, F. H. and Kools, J. A. (1969a). "Disfluency Behaviour of Elementary School Stutterers and Nonstutterers: Loci of Instances of Disfluency." *J. Speech Hear. Res.*, **12**, 308–318.

Williams, D. E., Melrose, Barbara and Woods, C. L. (1969b). "The Relationship Between Stuttering and Academic Achievement in Children." *J. Comm. Dis.*, **2**, 87–98.

Winkelman, N. W., Jr. (1954). "Chlorpromazine in the Treatment of Neuropsychiatric Disorders." *J. Am. Med. Assoc.*, **155**, 18–21.

Wischner, G. J. (1950). "Stuttering Behaviour and Learning: a Preliminary Theoretical Formulation." *J. Speech Hear. Disorders*, **15**, 324–335.

Wischner, G. J. (1952). "An Experimental Approach to Expectancy and Anxiety in Stuttering Behaviour." *J. Speech Hear. Disorders*, **17**, 139–154.

Wolpe, J. (1958). "Psychotherapy by Reciprocal Inhibition." Stanford University Press, California.

Wolpe, J. (1969). "The Practice of Behaviour Therapy." Pergamon Press, New York.

Yates, A. J. (1963). "Delayed Auditory Feedback." *Psychol. Bull.*, **60**, 213–232.

Young, M. A. (1961). "Predicting Ratings of Severity of Stuttering." *J. Speech Hear. Disorders., Monogr. Suppl.*, **7**, 31–54.

AUTHOR INDEX

Numbers in italics refer to the pages on which the references are listed in full.

SUBJECT INDEX